Cognitive-behavioral Psychotherapy for Anxiety

Hans-Christian Kossak

Cognitive-behavioral Psychotherapy for Anxiety

Brief Therapy with Hypnosis—The Practical Guide

Springer

Hans-Christian Kossak
Psychologischer Psychotherapeut
Bochum, Nordrhein-Westfalen, Germany

Foreword by
O. Berndt Scholz
Köln, Nordrhein-Westfalen, Germany

ISBN 978-3-662-69098-7 ISBN 978-3-662-69099-4 (eBook)
https://doi.org/10.1007/978-3-662-69099-4

This book is a translation of the original German edition "Kognitiv-behaviorale Psychotherapie von Ängsten" by Hans-Christian Kossak, published by Springer-Verlag GmbH, DE in 2020. The translation was done with the help of an artificial intelligence machine translation tool. A subsequent human revision was done primarily in terms of content, so that the book will read stylistically differently from a conventional translation. Springer Nature works continuously to further the development of tools for the production of books and on the related technologies to support the authors.

This Springer imprint is published by the registered company Springer-Verlag GmbH, DE, part of Springer Nature.
The registered company address is: Heidelberger Platz 3, 14197 Berlin, Germany

For my deceased wife and best friend

With great gratitude
for your patience, support
and unconditional love over so many
decades.

I do not treat anxiety.

I treat
Mrs. Maier or Mr. Müller
with their anxiety.

Foreword

Hypnotherapy has numerous interested parties both on the patient side and among those who apply it. Anyone who picks up literature and also "looks beyond the horizon" not only deepens their knowledge, but in the best sense of the word, practices scientific practice.

That hypnotherapists have long integrated established psychotherapeutic methods is by no means new. Psychoanalysis or Neuro-Linguistic Programming can be mentioned as examples. Working in trance is their greatest common denominator. Until the beginning of the millennium, behavior therapy struggled to systematically apply its extensive arsenal of methods in the hypnotherapeutic context. In the course of the so-called third wave, methods working with trance found their way into the superstructure of behavior therapy. The excellent book by Kirn et al. (2015)[1] is an impressive example of this. However, it only tentatively refers to the methodological breadth of hypnotherapy. This is already made clear by the title of the book.

Kossak presents a monograph in which both methodological approaches, hypnotherapy and behavioral therapy, are integrated in practice.

A new Psychotherapist Act has recently become universally binding. The guidelines formulated therein are so significant that even the study plans in the Master's program in Clinical Psychology and Psychotherapy at universities had to be reformulated. Imagine if a module on hypnotherapy had been included in the curriculum of this course. What breadth in training and research would hypnosis have experienced in its various forms and practical applications in a relatively short time! It is unfortunate that the boards of German hypnosis societies have missed a unique opportunity to emerge from the shadow existence of evidence-based hypnotherapy.

Why is this dictum pointed out and what does it have to do with Kossak's latest opus? The present book fills a gap in the intention to teach the combination of hypnosis and behavioral therapy. It is a refresher of basic knowledge for experienced practitioners who want to integrate behavioral therapeutic methods into

[1] Kirn T, Echelmeyer L, Engberding M (2015) Imagination in Behavior Therapy. Springer, Berlin, Heidelberg.

their hypnotherapeutic work—and vice versa. On the other hand, it can be a welcome suggestion for doctors and dentists who already work hypnotherapeutically and primarily treat patients with fears and phobias. And finally, the book can be a welcome guide for psychotherapists in training.

Often, moments of realization occur when the same facts are linguistically translated from one method to another. As an example, the linguistic transfer of cognitive restructuring into reframing or progression into hypnosis can be mentioned. The reader will have several such moments of realization while reading the book, as the majority of it consists of learning theory, behavioral therapy, and hypnotherapy explanations.

Likewise, the reader is repeatedly referred to basic literature according to the motto "Back to the roots!". This, of course, comes at the expense of new and latest literature.—A comparison with other (primarily behavior therapy) short-term therapies is missing. After all, the author's aim is to explain the approach he has developed and to illustrate it with practical case examples.

The author has a clear, unadorned diction. As a result, the text has a high information density in places. This is compensated by repeating various information in different contexts, according to the thesis "Repetitio est mater sapientiae".

All in all, it is to be hoped that the book will find a wide readership and, in particular, that the treatment concept developed by the author will be extensively applied. Otto Bernhardt Scholz, Universität Bonn

O. Berndt Scholz
University of Bonn

Preface

The innovation of the presented method includes that a complex short-term psychotherapy was developed and tested in practice here, which is based on extensive results of therapy research in behavior therapy, especially cognitive-behavioral therapy and experimental and clinical hypnosis, and relies on long experience and testing.

The aim of the book is to present a very effective *brief therapy* for anxiety, which is relatively quick to learn for skilled professionals and can actually be carried out within a session—and is permanently successful.

The book is intended to be informative for both beginners in the field of behavioral therapy or hypnosis and for advanced learners, and to motivate them to apply the method.

The combination of methods from cognitive-behavioral therapy and hypnosis is so far rarely used, but is very quickly understandable.

A short form can tempt you to apply it quickly without sufficiently mastering its entire foundations in theory and practice. For this reason, repetitions are listed under various aspects.

Therefore, in **Part I—The Basics**—in Chaps. 1 to 7 the fundamentals of both hypnosis, anxiety, and behavioral theories are presented in their basic principles, combined with a number of practical examples. However, they can hardly replace textbooks in these areas. The presentations of neuropsychology in these three areas are intended to contribute to their overarching understanding. They serve as a review for advanced learners and as introductions for beginners in the respective areas.

In **Part II—The Combinations**, the methods of cognitive behavioral therapy (CBT) relevant to the treatment of anxiety are primarily introduced in their basic principles in Chaps. 8 and 9. The focus is on the connection of CBT with the methods of hypnosis. For a better understanding, this chapter in particular is dealt with very extensively and is entirely practice-oriented.

The **Part III—The Practice—The Case Seminar** presents in Chap. 10 the diagnostic prerequisites for the application of the therapy method. Chapter 11 describes in great detail and also practically the four phases of short-term therapy with their individual steps, so that they can be understood relatively quickly in order to be applied soon. Chapter 12 is designed as a *practical case seminar*.

It provides vivid information with its *16 case presentations* about the diagnostics, indication, and implementation of the method. For this purpose, a special selection of different cases is available, each containing different diagnoses for the genesis of anxiety, and associated with it, differentiated therapeutic approaches or modifications.

The cases are presented as concisely as possible in their essential passages on anxiety. This enables readers to more easily understand the individual considerations and practical steps. In particular, Case 8 (Sect. 12.3.1) and Case 19 (Sect. 12.3.9) are very detailed and commented on to clearly illustrate the approach.

The *study questions* in the case documentation involve the readers and are intended to encourage them to make considerations as they are relevant in the system of short-term therapy of cognitive-behavioral hypnotherapy. They are then answered immediately. If these questions are too simple, then you as a reader are already advanced in CBT or hypnosis and simply skip these—or see them as confirmation of your considerations.

Then, in Chap. 13 the effects reported spontaneously by the patients are reproduced. They are followed by considerations on further possible applications of short-term therapy—and also thoughts on possible methodological limits.

Ultimately, Chap. 14 provides space for the presentation of the cautions, limitations, and contraindications of the method. The effectiveness of the method and its range of application are very high—measured by the numerous successful treatments, however, it should still be statistically proven.

Since the book is designed as a *practical guide*, even the theoretical parts often contain practical advice; in total, 27 cases are presented. The *case presentations* are numbered, making it easier to find and compare them when they are cited in several chapters. It should not go unmentioned that all case demonstrations come from real therapy sessions. Their presentations are anonymized in such a way that they do not allow any conclusions to be drawn about the respective person.

When a series of facts is to be enumerated, they are usually presented in a more tabular form. This prevents long and unmanageable sentences and promotes the desired learning processes. This is also served by the different *inserted boxes and highlights,* in which special facts such as practical tips, cases or examples are pointed out, as well as the total of 22 illustrations and 6 tables.

In this book, the male form was almost always chosen for therapist and patient. Fully aware of always including and addressing both, the form chosen here served to simplify the grammar and facilitate the presentation and understanding of the text.

Bochum Hans-Christian Kossak
October 2020

Acknowledgment

My thanks go to the many patients who have entrusted me with their life stories over the past many decades. Through them, I was able to gather my experiences in psychotherapy, especially with regard to my short-term therapy with hypnosis, which I was able to use both in the theoretical parts as well as in the case presentations.

Special thanks here to the clients Mrs. S. and Mrs. W., who spontaneously agreed to a recording of their therapy session; these are detailed here as Case 8 and Case 19.

I would now like to express my gratitude to Ms. Monika Radecki, Senior Editor at Springer Publishing. We have known each other through my authorship activities for at least thirty years. In a phone call with her, I mentioned the idea for this book. She spontaneously encouraged me to make this effective method of psychotherapy accessible to as many professional colleagues as possible. As usual, she advised me on the many questions that an author faces when completing his work.

I would also like to thank Mrs. Hiltrud Wilbertz for her numerous highly valued pieces of advice and the publishing support. She guided me safely through the diverse formatting pitfalls and requirements of modern electronic text processing. In doing so, she always maintained patience and calm, and continued to provide good advice on my many questions about text processing and text design, which an author needs for the latest computer and text processing tricks.

I am very grateful to Prof. Dr. O. Bernd Scholz for his extensive foreword and especially for his recommendations for additions and changes to the manuscript. They have contributed to the rounding off or sharpening of various presentations. His opinion as a well-known hypnosis researcher and hypnotherapist was particularly valuable to me in this regard.

My thanks now also go to Dr. med. dent. Gisela Zehner. We have been friends for many decades over hypnosis, and we had a very good human and professional collaboration on our joint book "Hypnose beim Kinder-Zahnarzt - Hypnosis in Pediatric Dentistry" published by Springer-Verlag (2011). She read my book manuscript in detail and very critically. Many thanks for the many helpful suggestions and impulses.

Thanks to Hans-Joachim Wolf, senior teacher i. R., with whom I have been friends for 66 years. As a Germanist and educator, he has expertly corrected my manuscript.

My English friend Peter Stephenson helped me to find the appropriate linguistic subtleties. Many thanks for this intensive support.

Ultimately—as always—my heartfelt thanks to my wife Silke. She calmly accepted my new manuscript when I spoke of four months of editing, also read the manuscript for correction, and advised me on text design. Now, after ten months had been reached due to the many text processing barriers, she also accepted that, knowing that it is important to me to share my practical experience with a hypnosis short therapy with psychotherapists and psychotherapists through this book.

Contents

About the Author

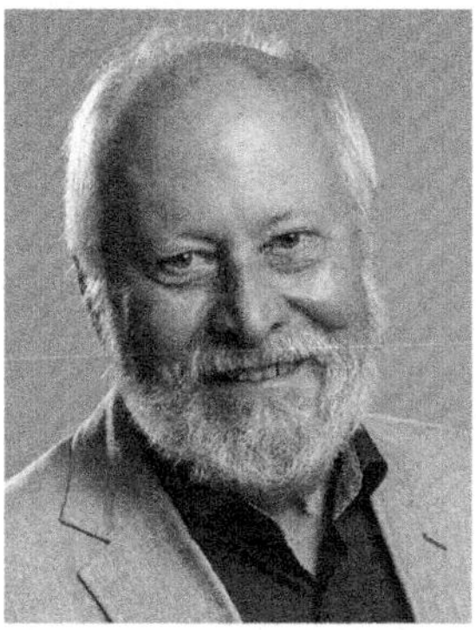

Dr. Hans-Christian Kossak, Dipl.-Psych., Psychological Psychotherapist and Child and Adolescent Counceling Psychotherapist with training certificates in Behavioral Therapy, Psychotherapy, Hypnotherapy.

Study of Psychology, University of Münster; seminars as a lecturer at the Ruhr University Bochum (Clinical Psychology), doctorate on the theory and combination of hypnosis and modern behavior therapy at the University of Bremen (Cognitive Psychology).

From 1969 to 2005, head of the Catholic Counseling Center for Education and Family Issues, Caritas Association for Bochum e. V.; there, founder of "Pluspunkt", the specialist therapy center for children and adolescents who are threatened or affected by disability.

Main areas of work: anxieties, psychosomatics, learning and performance disorders—and of course hypnosis applications in these areas. He is the founder of psychotherapy in the combination of cognitive behavioral therapy and modern hypnosis.

Continues to work as a lecturer and trainer of psychotherapists in hypnosis and behavioral therapy; lecturer for pediatric dentistry at the Berlin Dental Association. Speaker at national and international professional congresses. Author of numerous scientific professional publications and specialist books in his field.

1 A Brief Introductory Story

Almost everyone has experienced intense anxiety at least once in their life, whether it be while driving, during an accident, in a challenging situation, before a medical procedure, or before an examination. Therefore, most people are familiar with the sensation of fear and its accompanying symptoms. Sometimes, the experience of fear is so intense that it continues to evoke unpleasant memories when triggered by certain keywords or images. Many individuals have developed coping strategies over time to prevent the recurrence of such anxiety or reminders of it.

If an event is particularly traumatic, or if personal coping mechanisms are insufficient, the fear can persist. This fear can be so intense that it is perceived as life-threatening in certain situations, limiting the individual's behaviour and reducing their quality of life. Those affected may feel helpless, ashamed, and desperate. In such cases, the anxiety has become pathological and requires therapy, specifically psychotherapy.

Due to the widespread prevalence of anxiety disorders, their relatively high occurrence, the risk of chronicity and comorbidity, they result in work absences and high costs within the health system (Narrow et al. 2002).

Almost all therapeutic approaches have addressed the treatment of fears and have achieved varying degrees of success with their methods, each with its specific limitations.

Psychotherapy with Behavioural Therapy

Wolpe (1961) was the first to use behavioural therapy in the treatment of anxieties. Since about 1970, behavioural therapy (BT) with its various methods has also been used in Germany for the treatment of anxiety. Its further development over the last decades is cognitive behavioural therapy (CBT). It is the so-called second wave of behavioural therapy. Scientific therapy comparison studies show that CBT, in particular, has significantly higher effect sizes in the treatment of anxiety disorders and panic disorders than other treatments (e.g., Barlow 2002).

H.-C. Kossak, *Cognitive-behavioral Psychotherapy for Anxiety*,
https://doi.org/10.1007/978-3-662-69099-4_1

Consequently, the availability of therapy and literature on this subject has grown rapidly.

Parallel to this, in the 1970s, hypnosis experienced a renaissance in Germany and further developed as modern clinical hypnosis (Kossak 1991).

Psychotherapy with Behavioural Therapy Combined with Hypnosis
I soon discovered that the combination of BT and hypnosis represents a very effective therapy option. I published several articles on this, held seminars, and wrote my textbook on hypnosis (Kossak 1989). I also explored the then newly emerged cognitive-behavioural therapy, which was immediately relatively familiar to me, as it shared numerous elements with hypnosis. This led me to develop special cognitive-behavioural hypnotherapies for different disorders. This development towards imagination and hypnosis was only named as the third wave of BT much later.

Predominantly in the area of treatment of anxiety disorders, I was then able to condense the method to a short form so that it can be successfully and permanently applied by an experienced professional in psychotherapy or hypnosis within a brief hour, including diagnostics, therapy planning, hypnosis induction, relaxation, hypnotherapy, and follow-up discussion.

Further Developments
In the meantime, scientifically based hypnosis societies have formed worldwide from the beginnings mentioned above, with—in Germany alone—a total of over a thousand members. Basic and therapy research have increased both domestically and abroad and have produced an immense number of serious results about the effect and explanation of hypnosis. The scientific evidence of the psychotherapeutic method of hypnotherapy has long been extensively researched and documented with extensive studies (e.g., Revenstorf 2006). The effectiveness and efficiency of hypnosis is also confirmed in the medical field for certain diseases (Hefner 2010; Wark 2008), such as acute and chronic pain, which represents both a somatic and a psychological problem (e.g., meta-analysis by Montgomery et al. 2000). Associated with this, the publications of hypnosis specialist literature and also the specialist books on the treatment of fears with different cognitive-behavioural methods quickly increased (e.g., Chapman 2006; Wells 2011; Becker and Margraf 2016). Their combination with hypnosis for the treatment of fears was usually only briefly treated (e.g., Kirsch et al. 1999; Alladin 2008; Elkins 2017).

In the first edition of the aforementioned textbook (Kossak 1989), the treatment of fear using a *short form* of hypnosis and Cognitive Behavioural Therapy (CBT) is discussed. I further refined this approach over the years and presented it at seminars and national and international hypnosis congresses. The success with demonstration patients was swift, mirroring individual therapies, and remained permanent, with follow-up periods of up to 45 years. Numerous participants emailed me or spontaneously approached me during congress or event breaks because they were former clients or had also successfully tested my short therapy method as therapists (Kossak 2013).

This encouraged me to document the method after many successful cases and years, resulting in the present book. The focus here is on Cognitive Behavioural Therapy with hypnosis (CBTH).

The therapy successes remained consistent over the long observation periods. Although there were occasional minor changes, the basic framework remained intact—despite newer theoretical approaches—adhering to the motto "Never change a winning team".

Based on my experiences as a lecturer in training and further education seminars, the therapy method consciously relies heavily on the basic concepts of CBTH. This makes it relatively quick to learn for professionals such as doctors, psychotherapists, and dentists. I have tried to follow Albert Einstein's advice in this regard, as well as in psychotherapy sessions: "Things should be made as simple as possible. But not simpler."

Data analyses show that hypnosis as a therapy method for certain anxiety disorders (codable in ICD-10) is a highly effective therapy procedure and is just as effective as Cognitive Behavioural Therapy (Flammer 2006). Through the therapy steps outlined in this book, and with the promoted combination of both therapy methods, a surprisingly quick and permanently stable resolution of the anxiety problem occurs. Therefore, it is reasonable to assume that CBTH will soon also pass the effectiveness tests of science.

Increasing Therapy Demand

The demand for psychotherapy has significantly increased in the practices of psychotherapists, psychiatrists, psychologists, and doctors. Treatments with hypnosis are also increasingly in demand among dentists. In general, people are increasingly mentally burdened, resulting in long waiting times until the start of psychotherapy. This has led to the consideration of telephone or video therapy sessions, or even the demand for computer-assisted therapy programs.

Therefore, health insurance companies have been offering bonus payments since 2020 for the application of short therapy (SGB V, § 87 paragraph 2c; PTK-Newsletter of the Psychotherapists' Chamber NRW 1/2020).

Especially in times of personal, health, and economic crises, different existential fears arise, leading to an enormously high need for advice and treatment.

For these bottlenecks in supply capacities, the short therapy program documented in this book is suitable for certain disorders, especially fears. It has already proven successful and permanently effective within one session.

References

Alladin A (2008) Cognitive hypnotherapy. Wiley, Chichester

Barlow DH (2002) Anxiety and its disorders: the nature and treatment of anxiety and panic, 2. Aufl. Guilford Press, New York

Becker E, Margraf J (2016) Generalisierte Angststörungen. Beltz, Weinheim

Chapman RA (2006) The clinical use of hypnosis in cognitive behavior therapy. Springer, New York

Elkins GR (Hrsg) (2017) Handbook of medical and psychological hypnosis. Springer, New York

Flammer E (2006) Die Wirksamkeit von Hypnotherapie bei Angststörungen. Hypnose. Zeitschrift für Hypnose und Hypnotherapie 1(1+2):173–198

Hefner J (2010) Hypnose in der Medizin ist wirksam—Evident und Effizienz. Hypnose. Zeitschrift für Hypnose und Hypnotherapie 5(1+2):217–235

Kirsch I, Capafons A, Cardena-Buelna E, Amigó S (1999) Clinical Hypnosis and self-regulation. Cognitive perspectives. American Psychologists Association, Washington

Kossak H-C (1989) Hypnose. Psychologie Verlags Union, München

Kossak H-C (1991) Historische Entwicklung der Hypnose. Psychomed 3(3):157–159

Kossak H-C. (2013) Hypnose. Lehrbuch für Psychotherapeuten und Ärzte, 5. überarb. Aufl. Beltz, Weinheim

Montgomery GH, DuHamel KN, Redd WH (2000) A meta-analysis of hypnotically induced analgesia: how effective is hypnosis? Int J Clin Exp Hypn 48(2):138–153

Narrow WE, Rae DS, Robins LJ, Regier DA (2002) Revised prevalence based estimates of mental disorders in ther United States: using a clinical significance criterion to reconcile 2 surveys' estimates. Arch Gen Psychiatry 59(2):115–123

Revenstorf D (2006) Expertise zur Beurteilung der wissenschaftlichen Evidenz des Psychotherapieverfahren Hypnotherapie. Hypnose. Zeitschrift für Hypnose und Hypnotherapie 1(1+2):4–172

Wark DM (2008) What we can do with hypnosis: a brief note. Am J Clin Hypn 51(1):29–36

Wells A (2011) Kognitive Therapie der Angststörungen. Beltz, Weinheim

Wolpe J (1961) The systematic desensitization treatment of neuroses. J Nerv Ment Dis 112:189

Part I
The Basics

Hypnosis

After a historical introduction of hypnosis, the scientific facts for its delineation and definition follow. These include suggestions, hypnotizability, and its induction. The discussion includes free will in hypnosis and the requirements for the therapist.

In the section on neuropsychology, it is demonstrated through which mechanisms in the brain, control and filtering processes are possible with hypnosis.

Anxiety

After defining clinically significant anxiety and its forms, a seven-part model of the causation of anxiety is presented, which is particularly helpful for the practice of medical history collection and therapy planning.

Then, the neurophysiological and neuropsychological brain areas relevant to anxiety, along with their functions and networks, are introduced.

Behavioral Theory

The following are the fundamental paradigms of learning theory upon which Behavior Therapy is built. Using examples, the triggering and maintaining conditions of classical and cognitive behavioral theories are primarily illustrated in the context of fears.

Lastly, the neuropsychological factors and effect models are also presented here.

The reality is that,
what we perceive;
the truth does not always
agree with reality
(Buddhist Wisdom)

Hypnosis

2

Contents

H.-C. Kossak, *Cognitive-behavioral Psychotherapy for Anxiety*,
https://doi.org/10.1007/978-3-662-69099-4_2

The effects of hypnosis are likely based on inherent human abilities that were recognized thousands of years ago, such as in the treatment of pain or psychosomatic illnesses. Thus, modern treatment methods with hypnosis are also adapted to human abilities. Modern medical and psychological research has long recognized and demonstrated that numerous factors are effective, which can now be investigated and understood using modern scientific methods.

In this context, the effect of hypnosis on sensitive interpersonal aspects such as the therapist-patient relationship, their communication, and their expectation of the effect of hypnosis is crucial.

This chapter aims to demonstrate how much hypnosis is the subject of modern research, far removed from the prejudices of earlier times.

2.1 History of Hypnosis

Hypnosis has undergone numerous developments throughout history.

2.1.1 Historical Beginnings and Indigenous Peoples

What we refer to as *hypnosis* in our cultural circle today was already used in Chinese medicine 4000 years ago. Rites are also known among the Sumerians, the ancient Egyptians, and Indians that produce something akin to "sleep," in which the teacher or priest can then penetrate the soul of the person concerned to give instructions (e.g., Eliade 1960). In ancient Greece, priests in the Asclepieia, a type of medical center, induced a healing sleep. Many indigenous peoples of the present day still use similar procedures or applications for healing.

All these methods similar to hypnosis have commonalities • A social consensus in the culture or subculture about a disease model, i.e., about the origin and treatment of diseases.
- Belief in the ability of the healer and his ritual.
- Expectation of the healer—usually built up by the healer and then culturally handed down.
- Application of certain initiation techniques to bring about a changed (healing) experience. These introductions are usually ritualized by e.g., rhythmic activities (singing, dancing, prayer), sensory deprivation (perception narrowing), sight of a fixation point, fatigue, meditation, breathing techniques, drugs.

These latter aspects in particular can be found in many religious ceremonies such as in Zen Buddhism or in repetitive prayers like the rosary prayer or similar.

The effect is usually attributed to the ritual and its leader or the associated higher power such as spirit, God, etc. Later, representatives of these procedures can be found with modified methods as "healers" at fairs, as fakirs, magicians, bathers or tooth pullers.

2.1.2 From Enlightenment to Romanticism

Enlightenment
During the *Age of Enlightenment*, people began to seek scientific explanations for various phenomena. Franz Anton Mesmer (1735–1815) initially attributed these effects to the *magnetism* of living beings (also known as animal magnetism) and achieved great success with it, leading to a "magnetism fever" where almost all objects, including trees, were magnetized. Consequently, the healing successes of magnetizing, later referred to as mesmerizing, were significant in both individual and group treatments. Later, he referred to this force as a physical *fluidum*.

As the method quickly achieved success in healing diseases, it stimulated researchers to investigate its active factors.

James Braid (1795–1860), a Scottish eye surgeon, experimented with the method and found that the eye fixation on a shiny object triggered a state of drowsiness, which he termed "brain anemia". Due to this strong external resemblance to sleep, Braid (1843) named the state "hypnosis"—after the Greek god of sleep, *Hypnos*. He adopted this term from Simon Mialle (1826), but it was subsequently attributed to him and retained.

Shortly thereafter, Hippolyte Bernheim (1840–1919), Professor of Internal Medicine in Nancy, recognized that this behavior was not merely imagination or the effect of external powers, but was caused by suggestions, i.e., specific word formulations used to transform a thought into an action (Bernheim 1917).

Romanticism

Parallel to the scientific interest, during the era of Romanticism, magnetism and the behaviors achieved with it became very interesting for many of its representatives, such as C.W. Hufeland, W.F. Hegel, F.W.J. von Schelling, and Novalis (Friedrich Leopold Freiherr von Hardenberg). This interest in the *devided consciousness* was explored and dealt with in significant literary works by authors like E.T.A. Hoffman and E.E. Poe (Kossak 1999).

2.1.3 Beginning of Modern Research

Hypnosis research in the 19th century began to employ scientific methods beyond purely philosophical approaches. Notably, Heidenhain (1834–1897) discovered in his experiments that stimulus monotony plays a significant role in the initiation of magnetism (Heidenhain 1880). His students, the Soviet Russian Ivan Petrovich Pavlov and the Swiss Ludwig Binswanger and his assistant Oskar Vogt, are among the most important modern researchers.

In our timeline, we encounter Jean-Martin Charcot (1825–1893), who predominantly found hypnosis in hysterical patients. For him, hypnosis was abnormal behavior, a pathological state. It is very likely that his assistants, eager to please their boss, prepared the patients accordingly.

The intern of Bernheim and Charcot, Sigmund Freud (1856–1939), together with his friend, the internist Josef Breuer (1842–1925), successfully applied hypnosis to the patient Anna O., who was suffering from convulsions (Breuer and Freud 1895). In doing so, he recognized that physical diseases can have psychological causes, and thus became the founder of psychotherapy. Unfortunately, he was not adept at hypnotizing and stopped using hypnosis for various personal reasons, as it did not treat the causes. Regrettably, many of his students over several generations adopted this misjudgment.

Prohibition, Interdiction and Command suggestions

According to the understanding of the time about the origin of diseases, the treatment with hypnosis was purely symptom-oriented. This was particularly the case for diseases later defined as psychosomatic or psychological. This was compounded by hierarchical thinking and the associated authoritarian style in education, politics, and medicine. Therefore, in hypnosis treatment, patients were primarily addressed very authoritatively and given prohibition suggestions *("From now on you will no longer ...")* or command suggestions *("From now on you will ...").*

2.2 Natural Science—Hypnosis Research—Theories

With the increasing use of scientific research methods in medicine and psychology, we encounter I.P. Pavlov (1923) again, who in Russia laid the foundation for explanatory models of hypnosis (see Chap. 6). In the USA, T.X. Barber, who performed show hypnosis as a student to earn money, sought to understand the underlying principles through numerous controlled experiments (1958, 1969). Many researchers have followed in his footsteps, representing his cognitive-behavioral and social-cognitive theories.

Over time, representatives from other schools of thought, such as psychoanalysis, social psychology, and dissociation theory, have also contributed research and explanatory models from their perspectives.

This has resulted in a comprehensive field of research that, due to technological advancements, now employs MRI and can increasingly provide descriptions of the neurophysiological and neuropsychological effects of hypnosis. With each new research result, we gain more knowledge; however, this also leads to more questions and experiments. This is evidenced by the number of specialist articles and books on the subject, which alone registered a total of 2200 contributions in the database *pubmed* e.g. in the years from 2000 to 2010, of which over 400 are reviews.

2.3 Hypnosis in Clinical Practice

Due to the increasing and confirmed knowledge about the factors and mechanisms of hypnosis, it is now being used more frequently and successfully in psychotherapy, dentistry, and predominantly in psychosomatic medicine. Accordingly, hypnosis is officially recognized as a scientifically backed treatment: in England, it has been a fixed part of training for clinical professions since 1952, and in the USA since 1961. The *International Society of Hypnosis*, founded in 1958, is considered the umbrella organization of the later hypnosis societies.

Training

In German-speaking countries, hypnosis training is offered to professionals approved for clinical professions such as doctors, dentists, psychologists, and psychotherapists by scientifically based German-speaking hypnosis societies, for example by:

Milton Erickson Society (M.E.G.), Société Médicale Suisse d´Hypnose/ Swiss Medical Society for Hypnosis (SMSH), German Society for Hypnosis and Hypnotherapy e.V. (DGH), Austrian Society for Applied Depth Psychology and General Psychotherapy (ÖGATAP), German Society for Dental Hypnosis (DGZH), Milton Erickson Society Austria (MEG-Austria), German Society for Medical Relaxation Methods, Hypnosis, Autogenic Training and Therapy (DGÄHAT), Milton Erickson Society Austria, (MEGA), Austrian Society for Scientific Hypnosis (ÖGWH). They represent corresponding ethical, professional, and scientific standards (Hypnosis 2019, p. 232).

2.4 Research Results and Definitions

From the brief historical presentations, it is evident that there is extensive research on hypnosis, which produces very different results depending on the school of thought and provokes lively discussion.

For our purpose, to introduce a specific cognitive-behavioral treatment method with hypnosis, we will proceed pragmatically and use short versions of definitions, which are useful for the presentation and understanding of hypnosis and the treatment outlined here, in the following part.

2.4.1 What is Hypnosis?

In older case reports and scientific studies, hypnosis is not always precisely defined, making it difficult to compare statements about its effects. Based on these findings, more exact guidelines for its representation have been developed (Hagl 2019).

2.4.1.1 The Term "Hypnosis"

The term "hypnosis" can refer to three therapeutic approaches and additionally, a description of phenomena. Detailed explanations of these terms will be presented later in Chap. 9 on the practice of short-term therapy.

2.4.1.2 Terms Related to "Hypnosis"

2.4.1.2.1 Hypnosis as an Induction Method = Hypnosis Induction

Hypnosis induction is a specific procedure or initial ritual, which achieves hypnosis as a form of relaxation. Effective factors include a generally monotonous stimulus situation from the environment and the therapist's voice, and a narrowing of perception. The client should focus their perception more and more, thereby perceiving their own body processes such as breathing more, in order to finally deeply relax. (For detailed presentations, see Sect. 11.1.1).

2.4.1.2.2 Hypnosis as a Relaxation Method = Rest Scene

Following the hypnosis induction, the therapist guides the client's imagination towards a pleasant image, usually a landscape. The goal is to induce as deep a relaxation as possible after the introduction, in which the client feels comfortable and safe. (For detailed explanations and instructions, see Sect. 11.1.2.)

2.4.1.2.3 Hypnosis as a Therapy Method = Hypnotherapy

The third phase is the therapy phase, which follows the introduction and relaxation. In this phase, certain therapy and hypnosis methods are applied according to the diagnosis.

2.4.1.2.4 Hypnosis as a Form of Experience = Hypnosis Phenomena, Behaviour in Hypnosis

The form of experience refers to behaviour in hypnosis, which mainly occurs in phase three. This includes altered perception like hallucination, reduced pain perception, altered sense of time, physiological changes, etc. (A comprehensible description is given by the client in Sect. 12.3.12, Case 19, in the debriefing, therapy step 18.)

Since these terms are not always clearly separated, even in some publications, they are illustrated in Fig. 2.1. Here it becomes particularly clear that hypnosis is not synonymous with relaxation. Relaxation is merely a phase of the overall process.

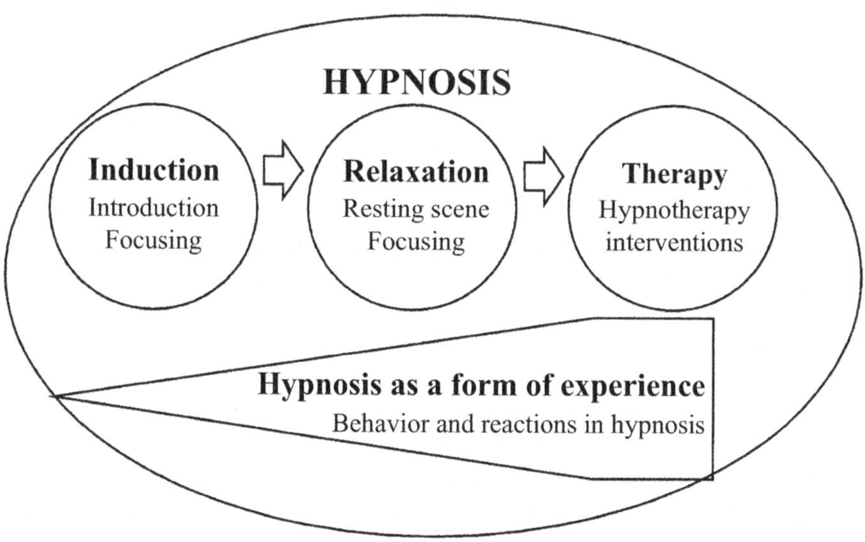

Fig. 2.1 The Terms Related to "Hypnosis"

2.4.2 Definition of Hypnosis

As previously illustrated, it is challenging to find a comprehensive definition of hypnosis due to its multifaceted nature and varying theoretical and research perspectives.

The discussion regarding the definition of hypnosis has been ongoing, starting with Hull (1933) and continuing to this day. The definition can vary, which in turn, affects the definition of hypnotizability (Kirsch et al. 2011, see below).

Definition of Hypnosis
Among the numerous attempts, the universally applicable aspects are summarized below.

- The behaviour following the induction of hypnosis is typically referred to as a trance.
- Hypnosis is a social interaction in which one person (the hypnotist) gives instructions or suggestions to another person (the subject or patient).
- Through these suggestions, the subject is encouraged to have certain experiences, such as changes in perception, memory, and voluntary actions (Kihlstrom 1985).
- In hypnosis, the subject's ability to criticize is reduced. Consequently, the words of the suggestions are accepted, for example, to not perceive pain stimuli or to perceive them differently (e.g., alleviated). This includes, among other things, not evaluating or perceiving objects, people, physical states, or feelings, or perceiving them differently (hallucinating).
- In hypnosis, verbal information (suggestions) takes precedence over cognitive control (Kossak 2013).

2.4.3 Delineations

To avoid common misconceptions about hypnosis, clear delineations are necessary.

2.4.3.1 Sleep

- People under hypnosis often appear to be sleeping during the relaxation phase. Based on this superficial observation, the complex event was named after the sleep god *Hypnos*—and the traditionally inherited name was retained.
- In sleep, REM phases can be detected, reflex excitability is reduced, behaviour is not influenceable, and the EEG is sleep-typical—but not in hypnosis.

2.4.3.2 Relaxation

- Many methodsinduce relaxation, such as autogenic training, progressive muscle relaxation (Jacobson 1938) and various meditation techniques. Typical physiological parameters can be detected in these, as well as in hypnosis—provided we are discussing the relaxation phase (Vaitl 2020; Kossak 2020). Compared to general relaxation, the level of alertness decreases in highly suggestible individuals during hypnosis (Haipt et al. 2017).
- Hypnosis should not be equated with relaxation, because in the therapy phase following relaxation, post-traumatic experiences are reactivated and processed, which do not contain many elements of relaxation.

2.4.3.3 Everyday Behaviour

- In hypnosis, similar patterns can be observed in the EEG and in everyday behaviour when performing comparable actions or experiences.
- The forms of behaviour and experience shown in hypnosis can also be found in normal everyday life—only in hypnosis they are brought about more directly and quickly. Here the schools of thought differ. Behaviourist theories view hypnosis as something that can also be experienced under certain conditions in everyday life. In contrast, other theories propose that hypnosis involves an altered state of consciousness (Kirsch 2011).
- Hypnosis is also possible in complete wakefulness, for example in sports, to focus on the upcoming activity (tunnel vision) and to carry out the previously trained sequences almost reflexively with optimal arousal.

2.4.4 Forms of Hypnosis and Terminology

Numerous scientific results from various research directions suggest that there are not just one, but multiple forms of hypnosis (Weitzenhoffer 1989). However, these forms cannot yet be clearly separated and defined. Instead, they should be viewed as indicators of different results under similar conditions. Given that this is still a subject of scientific dispute, we will focus more on the currently recognized forms.

2.4.4.1 Autogenic Training

Autogenic training, developed by Schultz (1932) as a form of self-hypnosis (see below), is now a common relaxation method. Through formulaic intention formation and self-suggestions, relaxation occurs, leading to psychosomatic influence.

2.4.4.2 Self-hypnosis or Autohypnosis

The guided (see above) learned autohypnosis is used to independently induce relaxation and exercise self-control in relevant or impairing situations.

2.4.4.3 Heterohypnosis or Allohypnosis

This includes hypnosis induced under the guidance of another person (hetero), typically by a therapist.

2.4.4.4 Spontaneous Hypnosis

Spontaneous hypnosis occurs when certain triggering stimuli are present. This can happen after a posthypnotic task (see Sect. 3.6), such as *"When you see a dog, you react spontaneously with relaxation"*. With persistent monotonous sensory stimulation, hypnosis can occur spontaneously, as is possible with so-called highway hypnosis during long and monotonous road conditions.

2.4.4.5 Fractionated Hypnosis

If the hypnosis is interrupted (fractionated) by the therapist, the subsequent re-induction can lead to a deepening of relaxation (Vogt 1895a, b).

2.4.5 The Evolution of Modern Hypnosis

The indications and methods of hypnosis have evolved from magnetism to the present day.

2.4.5.1 Transition from Symptom Therapy to Causal Therapy

As previously demonstrated, therapy was traditionally focused directly on the symptom until the mid-20th century. With the advancement of scientific knowledge, it was increasingly discovered in various areas of medicine and psychotherapy that there are more or less clear causes for symptoms, diseases, or problems, which need to be investigated and treated, rather than merely addressing the symptom superficially.

> **Important**
> Modern hypnosis is applied causally, that is, it acts on the causes.

2.4.5.2 Transition from Authoritarian to Non-Directive Therapy

In addition, a new zeitgeist in communication, culture, education, and so on, developed parallel to this, which was an alternative to the previously authoritarian approach. Notably, Carl R. Rogers (1902–1987) developed the non-directive, client-centered therapy, in which the therapist-patient relationship is a determining factor. In this zeitgeist, Milton H. Erickson (1901–1980) developed a hypnosis application that requires a good patient-therapist relationship as a co-determining factor. Essential for his form of treatment in hypnosis are *indirect suggestions*, which improve cooperation and reduce resistance. This is supplemented by certain speech patterns and the use of resources offered by or inherent in the patient for change, to name just a few.

This differentiates itself from "other forms of hypnosis" through various methods, also known as "Ericksonian Hypnosis"; however, its effectiveness is comparable.

2.4.5.3 Is Hypnosis an Independent Therapy Method or an Adjunctive Method?

Almost consistently, many therapists, for example in the medical field, use hypnosis as an *adjunct*, that is, as an additional method (Kirsch et al. 1999; Hagl 2019).

The term *Hypnotherapy* can lead to the misconception that hypnosis is an independent type of treatment (Kirsch et al. 1999).

This means that a known and proven basic therapy such as psychoanalysis, behavior therapy, and so on, is combined with hypnosis, thereby optimizing application and increasing the effectiveness of therapy. This requires knowledge and training in both the basic therapy and hypnosis.

In contrast, in Ericksonian Hypnosis, it is largely believed that hypnosis can be considered an independent form of therapy. However, the theoretical scientific prerequisites—such as a theory of its own with its own disease, diagnosis, and therapy model—have not yet been met.

Regardless of this, hypnosis, when applied by a licensed professional, is recognized by health insurance as a therapeutic method.

2.4.6 The Cognitive-Behavioural Hypnosis Model

- In the cognitive-behavioural hypnosis model, hypnosis is viewed as an *adjunct method* for cognitive-behavioural interventions (imaginations, behaviour changes, approach, cognitive restructuring etc.) (Kirsch 1992).
- In this model, the construct of an *altered state of consciousness* is rejected.
- Its theoretical basis is formed by the fact that hypnosis brings about a change in the person's experiences and behaviours through hypnosis suggestions.
- The focus is on the social therapist-patient interaction, which is determined by expectations and belief systems. In this theoretical structure of cognitive-behavioural therapy (CBT), the subconscious does not play a significant role as a cause and solver of problems, which can be accessed (only) through hypnosis according to the state model (Chapman 2006).
- In the meta-analysis of 18 studies, the effectiveness of CBT with and without hypnosis combination was examined (Kirsch et al. 1995). According to this, the combination of CBT with hypnosis (CBTH) is the most effective therapy method, as the effects of both methods add up (e.g., Alladin and Alibhai 2007).

Practice and Theory

The numerous and very different hypnosis theories are of high academic-scientific interest, including the discussion of whether hypnosis is another state of consciousness. For the practicing therapist, the application of clinical hypnosis is primarily important. This is naturally determined by the therapist's respective therapy orientation and then more oriented towards e.g., psychoanalysis, ego-state therapy, or cognitive behavioural therapy (Heap 2001) and their opening to mindfulness (Orsillo et al. 2012).

2.5 The Basic Factors and Determinants of Hypnosis

Numerous factors are involved in the effectiveness of hypnosis with its variety of phenomena. Three areas are particularly significant (e.g., Mazzoni et al. 2013).

Three Main Factors for the Effectiveness of Hypnosis (see Fig. 2.2)

- The hypnosis suggestions
- The interindividual effectiveness of hypnotizability or susceptibility to respond to suggestions
- The induction process

2.5.1 Suggestion

In everyday communication, suggestion is associated with the application of a certain verbal skill, with which one exercises power and manipulation, to deceive

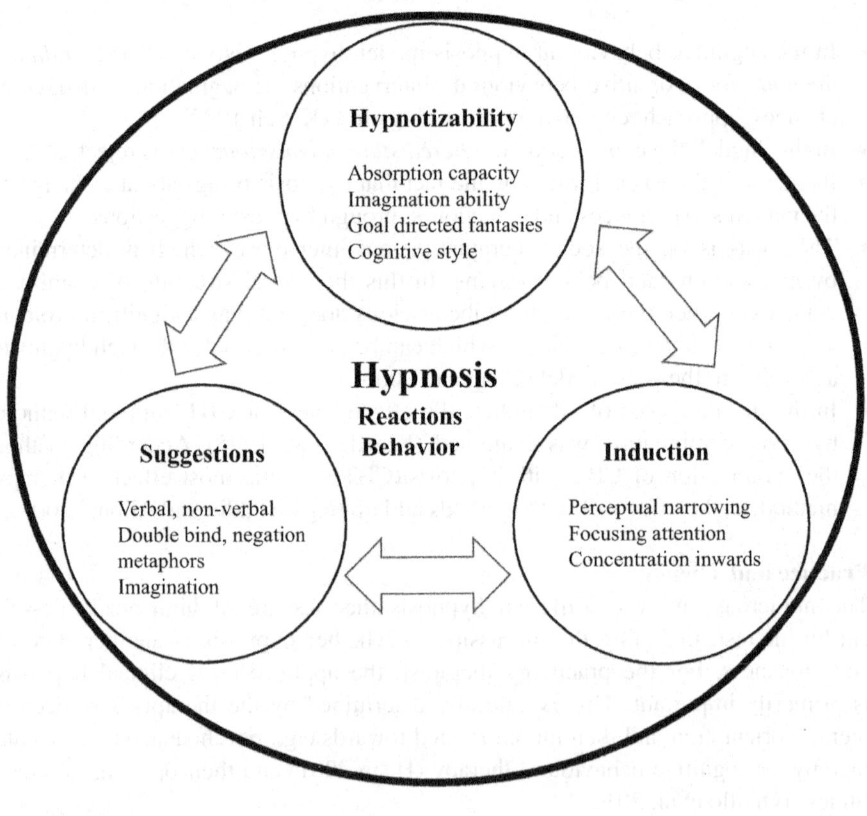

Fig. 2.2 The interaction of the components of hypnosis

another person, who is then referred to as foolish for allowing such a thing to happen.

The suggestion referred to here is a form of *communication* in which alternatives are offered, thus maintaining freedom of choice. However, the intention is to achieve something else that then eludes conscious control (Gheorghiu 1987, 1996, 2000). For example, it includes the double-bind suggestion "*Do you want to relax moderately, lightly, or deeply?*" The client can freely choose between these three options. However, the suggestion implies that the client unknowingly decides to apply relaxation, regardless of its depth. This creates expectations such as "*relaxation will follow shortly*", which are then largely followed without reflection. Similarly, the suggestion: "*What has now changed positively*" directs the search that something must have changed positively (see Sect. 11.9).

Suggestions work particularly well when they are tailored to the client's reference system, such as in the rest scene. For this, the client's descriptions of his rest scene are explored and used to formulate suggestions for designing his personal hypnosis rest scene, combined with relaxation and well-being suggestions.

Hans Christian Andersen's novel "The Emperor's New Clothes" from 1835 serves as a classic example: Only those who are stupid or unfit for their office cannot see these clothes.

2.5.1.1 Suggestions without Hypnosis

It becomes clear that suggestions do not necessarily have to be associated with hypnosis. In everyday life, we encounter many non-verbal suggestions such as: certificates in the waiting room, status symbols like a car or Rolex watch, uniforms, etc. Placebos (dummy preparations) are also worth mentioning, to which one reacts in the announced manner, even with the associated side effects.

2.5.1.2 Negations as Suggestions

One is too quick to deny the unwanted and paradoxically achieves the opposite.

> **Denials highlight the denied**
> Denials can work like suggestions, by perceiving the denied feeling particularly highlighted.
>
> **Examples include:**
>
> *"You will have no fear in the exam"*
> *"You will have no pain"*
> *"Stand in front of a wall and think of no bear."*

This phenomenon is studied by psycholinguistics and has been experimentally proven: The denial causes the *paradoxical effect of thought suppression* (Wegner et al. 1987). This means that the denial creates a clear emphasis on the negated. This in turn means that the more effort is made to suppress the thought, the more persistently it remains (Trinder and Salkovskis 1994). Earworms can be an example of this.

Denials only formulate what should be omitted or ignored. They are often very generally formulated and additionally fix the attention even more on the negated. As a result, hardly any helpful strategies for future action can be derived.

2.5.1.3 Operationalizing Clear, Positive, and Goal-Oriented Instructions

Providing clear instructions on how to act or feel in the future enables the client to identify behavioural goals and act accordingly.

Examples of Positive/Goal-Oriented Suggestions

- For exam anxiety: "*You are well-prepared for your exam. You can relax quickly and effectively. Thus, you can approach the exam calmly and wait in a relaxed manner for the questions.*"
- For fear of dogs: "*You see the dog, can look at it calmly and remain calm (apply your relaxation), breathe easily and continue calmly.*"
- For amnesia of the number five: "*The number five will become indifferent to you.*"
- For switching off thoughts: "*Your thoughts come and go .... They will become indifferent to you over time.*"

Moreover, in conversations, such as explorations, the repeated repetition of a negation and the associated contents such as feelings, actions, and aversions become more prominent in the foreground of attention and are then imprinted more intensively. Therefore, concentrated conversations about fears can even intensify them. These negative topics should only be the focus of therapy as long as necessary. A change of topic then offers the chance to experience, perceive, etc., something else associated with it. In everyday life, this would be the abrupt distraction by changing topics and actions. ◄

► **Formulations of Instructions or Suggestions**

- Must be clear and unambiguous.
- Should only be positive.
- Should be short and manageable.
- Provide clear instructions on what exactly should be done (motorically, cognitively, emotionally, etc.).
- Are therefore goal-oriented and action-oriented.
- Are also effective when given indirectly.

For further details on communication, see Sect. 1.5.8.

2.5.2 Hypnotizability

Since the beginning of the experimental exploration of hypnosis, questions have arisen about which individuals are hypnotizable, whether it is perhaps an innate ability, and whether the reaction to hypnosis instructions is involuntary, voluntary, simulated, or courtesy reactions, etc.

2.5.2.1 Scientific Results

Based on numerous experiments and in accordance with various schools of thought, we can make the following statements:

- A distinction must be made between suggestibility and hypnotizability. Suggestions can be given without reference to hypnosis, for example, in the case of the double-bind: "*Do you want to put on the red or the green hat*?"
- This leads to challenges in defining and constructing tests that are intended to measure the responsiveness to hypnosis, i.e., hypnotizability (Braffman and Kirsch 1999).
- Ultimately, a pragmatic approach is adopted by presenting tasks to the test subjects or clients that require hypnotic behaviour, such as Item 9 of the HGSHS: A (Harvard Group Scale of Hypnotic Susceptibility Form A), the auditory hallucination of a fly (Shor and Orne 1962).
- The best-known and most widely used test is the *Stanford Hypnotic Susceptibility Scale* (SHSS) with 12 items. It was developed by Weitzenhoffer and Hilgard (1958), refined (as seen above in HGSHS), and has been translated and standardized into almost all common languages to this day. Across nations, languages, and cultures, very consistent results have been obtained so far.

Tests and Everyday Practice

Testing hypnotizability with various scales such as the SHSS primarily holds academic significance for experimental comparative data. In practice, this testing can be very time-consuming and may not provide more differentiated information than the patient's reaction to the induction and the suggestions of the rest scene (Woody and Sattler 2017). Rather, the therapist already receives information about the patient's cooperation in hypnosis through the reactions during the induction and the rest scene, which can then be pragmatically referred to and used as hypnotic cooperation ability.

2.5.2.2 Factors of Hypnotizability

There are clearly definable factors of hypnotizability.

People with high hypnotizability possess the following factors or abilities:

2.5.2.2.1 Absorption Ability

Individuals with absorption ability have a strong inwardly directed attention, are hardly distractible and primarily focused on the desired/agreed/suggested event. Other external or internal stimuli are then faded out. They only perceive the focused goal of their attention. In fact, highly hypnotizable individuals can engage so much in the hypnosis suggestions that they no longer perceive the world around them and are exclusively in the suggested world like "Green Meadow" or "I am sitting as a 6-year-old on my grandmother's lap, smelling her perfume, feeling her caress, hearing her voice etc."

Everyday example: An exciting or fascinating event (crime, football game, film, accident) can focus the involuntary attention on it so much that the perception of the environment fades into the background.

2.5.2.2.2 Imaginative Ability

Imagination, or imaginative ability, involves being able to vividly imagine situations or sensory impressions. This includes not only—as often thought—static images like e.g. "holiday or album photos". It is an ability to imagine impressions on almost all levels of perception or even to "really" experience them (Barber 1999). This includes—depending on the meaning and preference of the imaginations—the imagined perception of an otherwise real event or stimulus, i.e. experiencing something as real in hypnosis, such as the warmth on grandma's lap mentioned in the example above, the scent of the first kiss, the smell of fire at an accident etc. Some clients open their eyes after hypnosis, blink slightly disoriented and report e.g. that they just met their (deceased) grandmother or went for a walk in the town NN.

2.5.2.2.3 Goal-directed Fantasies

The imagination of a certain action can already cause the corresponding movements and physiological correlates. Therefore, not only the static imagination "arm", but the goal-directed fantasy "I lift the forearm to grab" has an effect.

2.5.2.2.4 Cognitive Style

Hypnotizability implies different cognitive styles (McConkey and Barnier 2004). Individuals with high hypnotizability have a *holistic thinking style,* i.e. a holistic cognitive processing (e.g. Crawford 1988). Specifically, it involves experiencing scenes given in hypnosis like "*You are sitting on your grandmother's lap*" as a holistic scene with all optical, haptic, gustatory etc. impressions.

Individuals with a more *analytical thinking style* find these complex experiences in hypnosis somewhat more difficult. They need more time to experience such a complex scene; they start from individual details suggested by the therapist and slowly put them together into a more complex experience.

For the hypnosis therapist, patients who experience holistically are of course helpful. They experience complex scenarios and act within them. However, this does not mean that those who think analytically show less successful imaginations or hypnosis reactions. They need to be slowly introduced to the complex event through the perception and experience of the details of the scene.

2.5.2.3 Hypnotizability, Personality, and Therapy Success

Research is being conducted to determine whether hypnotizability, which is influenced by several individual abilities, is associated with certain personality traits, whether it can be learned, or even whether it co-determines the success of therapy.

2.5.2.3.1 Personality Traits

- Hypnotizability does not correlate with any measurable personality factors such as extraversion/introversion or pathological personality traits, for example, neuroticism.
- Hypnotizability is primarily a stable factor that remains consistent even when measured over many decades.

2.5.2.3.2 Learnability

- Hypnotizability can only be influenced or conditioned under certain conditions, including positive expectations of hypnosis (Kirsch 2001), the high status of the hypnotist (De Vogue and Sachs 1973), or contingent biofeedback training of certain brainwave parameters (Wickramasekera 1971).

2.5.2.3.3 Gender, Health, and Hypnotizability

- Women tend to have higher values in both objective and subjective hypnotizability (Cardena et al. 2007).
- Highly hypnotizable individuals have fewer stress-related dysfunctions compared to those with low hypnotizability (Jambrik et al. 2005).

2.5.2.3.4 Therapy Success and Hypnotizability

- There is no significant correlation between hypnotizability and therapy success (Lynn et al. 2008). This suggests that even people with low hypnotizability can achieve good therapy results with hypnosis.

2.5.2.4 Therapy Success Even Without Hypnotizability

The aforementioned research result implies the following conclusion for everyday therapy: If a test for hypnotizability or the actual hypnosis situation reveals that a client does not respond well to hypnosis, therapists are then faced with the decision to continue or possibly stop. The latter would be detrimental for the client and would reflect the therapist's lack of flexibility or competence to deal with more challenging situations.

Even if a client has a limited imagination and is therefore poorly hypnotizable, they still have a right to competent treatment. It is up to the therapist to apply methods that require less or no imagination. Imagination training can also be carried out, starting with imagining an apple, for example (Kossak 2013, p. 347). The client may then understand what is meant by imagination and implement it mentally. They may also realize that they can "let go" into imaginations, as they previously associated being a softie, dreamer, or losing control of their feelings, which they had previously been able to hold back with effort. Alternatively or additionally, progressive muscle relaxation according to Jacobson (1938) or the telling of metaphors for relaxation would be recommended in such cases.

If a patient does not respond to all the aforementioned aids, the ultimate insight remains that hypnosis should not be applied in this case.

2.5.3 Induction—The Initiation Procedure of Hypnosis

The induction or initiation of hypnosis involves further building trust and relaxation. It is a ritual in which the patient increasingly focuses their attention and perception, thus directing their attention from external stimuli to their internal processes of breathing and relaxation. The goal is the deep relaxation of the patient, in which they follow the suggestions of the therapist. In doing so, they also accept suggestions that may not objectively correspond to their experiences or perceptions. This way of experiencing is usually referred to as a trance.

2.5.3.1 Suggestions for Induction—Effective Factors

- Credibility and safety of the therapist as a hypnosis expert
- Slow, monotonous, calming language
- The pitch of the voice should be lower according to relaxation and at a pleasant volume
- Clarity and comprehensibility of language
- Concreteness and imagery of the language (VAKOG, Sect. 2.5.8.4).
- Short sentences with many repetitions, very simple grammar
- Feedback of current events, i.e., if eye redness is observed, report the associated sensation as a suggestion: *"Your eyes are starting to burn and are getting more and more tired..."*

2.5.3.2 Methods of Induction

Some therapists believe that they need to be equipped with a variety of induction methods to achieve a successful induction. Accordingly, there are books that mainly deal with inductions and induction techniques. However, a basic repertoire of about two to four induction procedures can usually suffice. Therapists should gain extensive experience with these methods and possibly vary them to adapt them to the individual needs of the patient. By following the above recommendations, the therapist will be successful with their induction, quiet scene, and hypnosis conversation.

Ultimately, the therapist's confidence and credibility as a personality and as a hypnosis expert is probably decisive for good compliance. This is associated with confidence in handling the verbal "tools".

If, despite all therapeutic efforts, no induction is successful, then reference should be made to the limits that the patient or the method bring with them (see Chap. 12).

The suggestions for two induction methods are given in exact wording in Chap. 11 (intervention phases).

2.5.4 Hypnosis as a Relaxation Technique

Following the induction of hypnosis, the so-called *relaxation scene* is introduced.

The content of this scene is pleasant and calm, preferably drawn from the patient's own experiences. It should be explored before the start of the induction so that the scene contains as many elements as possible that the patient finds vivid and can then imagine in a trance. Even during the exploration of the relaxation scene, it can sometimes be observed that the patient communicates non-verbal signals about the scene, such as smiling or relaxed shoulders. This communication should then be used with appropriate word formulations for a relaxing effect. After a short time, the patient will then subjectively be in this relaxation scene and relax.

2.5.4.1 About the term *Relaxation Scene*

Sometimes the term relaxation*image* is used. However, the instruction of an image is more likely to be associated with something static like a photograph.

Since the patient in hypnosis can have multidimensional or multimodal experiences, perceptions and sensations, and even experience himself or others acting, the term relaxation*scene* (=rest scene) is more appropriate. This indirectly suggests the experience of a complex or moving scene.

Some therapists use the term *feel-good scene,* which also corresponds well to this dynamic.

2.5.4.2 Function of the *Relaxation Scene*

- *Relaxation* of the patient
- *Preparation* for the following interventions
- *Building trust* with the patient and his application of hypnosis
- *Safety:* if too stressful experiences occur during therapy, the patient can be offered to use the relaxation scene and relax there again.

Often, the already mentioned "Green Meadow" or "On the Beach" is chosen as the standard scene. However, it should also be explored which aspects of the area are particularly pleasant, such as a cliff in autumn or a flat beach in the Caribbean. In this way, each patient gets his subjectively relaxing relaxation scene.

The formulations for this are like those for the induction: slow, calm, VAKOG (see Sect. 2.5.8.2) used. During the relaxation scene, the therapist should continue to communicate verbally with the patient (= rapport), in order to receive feedback on the effectiveness of his suggestions and to reinforce them differentially or to modify his suggestions.

Only when the patient is sufficiently relaxed can the next therapeutic phase be initiated. The practical representations for this are shown in Chaps. 10 and 11, Therapy Phase 4.

2.5.5 Hypnosis as a Form of Experience—Behaviour in Hypnosis—The "Hypnosis Phenomena"

With the beginning of the relaxation in hypnosis (= trance), under the guidance of the therapist, suggestions are made which alter the patient's ways of experiencing. These changes are often referred to as phenomena of hypnosis. Of the numerous possibilities, only a few are mentioned here in keyword form (see Table 2.1).

This variety of experiential possibilities offers applications in numerous therapeutic areas. In our presentations, we limit ourselves to the application of hypnosis in the treatment of fears.

All the aforementioned behaviours have been extensively researched experimentally to explain their neurophysiological and neuropsychological effects, and then use them in therapy. Numerous experiments confirm the therapeutic effectiveness of hypnosis with its possibilities.

2.5.6 Depth of Hypnosis

In everyday language, we often say someone is "deeply away" while reading an exciting book or watching a film, or during hypnosis. This means being far removed from the current situation and deeply immersed in the experience: "*I was on the beach of NN*" and not "*I imagined being on the beach of NN*".

Table 2.1 Behaviour in hypnosis and its relationship to anxiety therapy, so-called phenomena of hypnosis/trance phenomena in anxiety treatment

Behaviour in Hypnosis: General Description	Relevance for Anxiety Treatment: Examples
Motor Reactions: Catalepsy, Ideomotor	Response prevention = Prevention of avoidance behaviour
Psycho-physiological Changes: Relaxation, Cardiovascular, Temperature, Immune System, Histamine, Adrenaline etc.	Relaxation—Counterconditioning Sensitization: for tension and relaxation; physiological processes
Changes in Memory and Time Perception: Amnesia, Age Regression, Time Distortion as Time Lapse or Slow Motion	Experience the time of tension (anxiety) as shortened Possibly experience the time without fear as in childhood
Hallucinations: Altered perception of objective stimuli	Perceive anxiety-triggering stimulus differently (=as neutral)
Changes in psychological Effects: Dissociation, Distraction, Posthypnotic Suggestions	Observe oneself from a changed perspective and experience without anxiety Redirect attention, away from fear Suggestion to relax and act without fear in the future

For a long time, attempts have been made to explore the depth of a hypnosis effect, and different experiments and questionnaires have been developed for this purpose. However, the experienced depth of relaxation or hypnosis is very difficult to measure objectively, i.e., to express numerically and thus process statistically. People react with their experiences extremely differently, so the attempt to use depth scales to measure hypnosis has hardly produced scientifically statistically usable results, especially since they caused numerous methodological problems and errors in the experimental design.

Can hypnosis and the depth of hypnosis be judged from the outside by observers? This again results in methodological errors, since a subjective experience (e.g., the hallucination of the scent of a rose) is hardly objectively observable from the outside. The readings derived from the EEG or similar possibly shows specific reactions; however, are these an indication of depth?

2.5.7 The Hypnosis Therapist

Historically, hypnosis therapists were believed to possess a certain power and ability to influence their patients. This belief dates back to centuries ago when priests, acting on behalf of the gods, were thought to have this power. Among indigenous peoples, it continues to be the shamans. Later figures such as Mesmer, Braid, and Freud, who corresponded to the healer image of their time, were also believed to possess a certain knowledge and power of the mind.

In his novel *Mario and the Magician* (1930), Thomas Mann portrays the hypnotist and magic artist Cipolla as an unsympathetic man who exercises power with hypnosis, imposes his will on his theatre guests, and even makes them act against their morals. Mann uses this character to foreshadow the rise of Hitler. Crime novels or comics featuring hypnosis often depict a similar power dynamic, portraying the hypnotist as superior. The hypnotist is often characterised by a piercing gaze, conjuring hand gestures, and short, concise suggestions such as: "*You are hypnotized, you are subject to my will*".

In line with the spirit of the times, Rogers and Skinner (1956) began to explore the therapist-patient relationship, a subject that remains a focus of research in medicine and psychology or psychotherapy today. In the field of hypnosis, it was T.X. Barber (1969) who began to explore this social relationship, a line of inquiry that continues to this day.

2.5.7.1 Generally Applicable Therapist Variables

Essential Variables

- There are no specific personality traits that characterize a good hypnotist, but rather a good therapist (Whitehead et al. 2008).
- Empathy, activity, attentiveness, warmth, communication skills, and authenticity are all important traits (Bergin and Lambert 1978).

- Competencies in the field are essential, i.e., appropriate training that imparts professional knowledge and skills, as well as the associated values and attitudes (Berven 1987).
- Hypnotizability is not a necessary trait for a hypnosis therapist. For example, one of my seminar participants achieved good effects as a therapist with the induction and rest scene for his patients, but could not experience it himself. This demonstrates that hypnosis is a clinical "tool" that requires professional competence, but not personal hypnotizability.

2.5.7.2 Specifics of a Hypnosis Session and Requirements for the Hypnotherapist

The following aspects are primarily based on Kossak (2013, p. 287 ff.).

- **Induction**: The initiation of hypnosis requires the therapist to have a concentrated perception of the patient's behaviour. The therapist must observe very carefully to precisely reinforce the behaviour aspects relevant to the induction of hypnosis (see Sect. 2.5.1).
- **Intimacy:** The hypnosis session represents a very intimate relationship. It is established by the very private question or problem posed by the patient and the associated anamnesis conversation. Added to this is the fact that the patient has his eyes closed from the induction of hypnosis.
- **Familiarity:** The situation creates a kind of familiarity and psychological as well as physical closeness, which makes it easier to address and work on problems. At the same time, this situation can also arouse the desire for greater closeness on both sides, which the therapist must handle professionally.
- **Reduction of attention and critical ability**: In hypnosis, the patient's attention is narrowed (see Sect. 3.1), associated with a selectively reduced critical ability towards external and internal stimuli (e.g., ambient noise; fear thoughts, see Sect. 3.1). This suggests that the patient's vulnerability in this situation is very high and therefore requires very sensitive handling.
- **Suggestions and Imaginations:** The suggestions and imaginations necessary for therapy must be well prepared to meet individual therapy goals; however, these are only successful if they include the patient's desires, experiences, and abilities.
- **Responsiveness:** During therapy, suggestions and imaginations often have to be formulated spontaneously. This requires professional knowledge, anamnesis knowledge, flexibility, and also life experience of the therapist to be able to react spontaneously.
- **Language communication:** Communication during the hypnosis session is largely through language, i.e., through the patient's reports about his feelings and the corresponding statements or suggestions of the therapist. This can only succeed if the therapist adapts to the patient's language and speaks carefully, briefly, and clearly.

- **Attitudes and expectations of hypnosis**: Depending on prior information from radio, television, or print media, patients' attitudes towards hypnosis vary: if they have seen show hypnosis or a scientific contribution to hypnosis, their expectations and fears will be very different. Accordingly, the therapist should be informed about this or ask his patients about it and clarify or inform them (Capafons et al. 2006). The treatment is more effective if the therapist adapts his approach to the patient's expectations and requirements (Lazarus 1973).
- **Multitasking of the therapist:** The therapist must—as in other therapies—convert the theory and the individual therapy steps derived from it into instructions or suggestions. In doing so, he must formulate the suggestions appropriate for the patient spontaneously, observe him in a differentiated manner, and react to the verbal, but especially the non-verbal signs he shows, and further process them in word formulations correcting or reinforcing etc. All of this must happen as spontaneously as possible and requires synchronous work on several cognitive and emotional levels, i.e., high concentration and imaginative ability of the therapist (Brown and Fromm 1986).
- **Therapist's confidence.** The therapist's confidence is of great importance for the desired patient reactions or cooperation. Only after that is the induction method a decisive factor (Wolberg 1982).

2.5.8 Communication in Hypnosis

After numerous significant variables and factors of the therapist-patient relationship have been mentioned, the question arises as to what is typical of hypnotic communication or how it can be practically implemented (see Fig. 2.3).

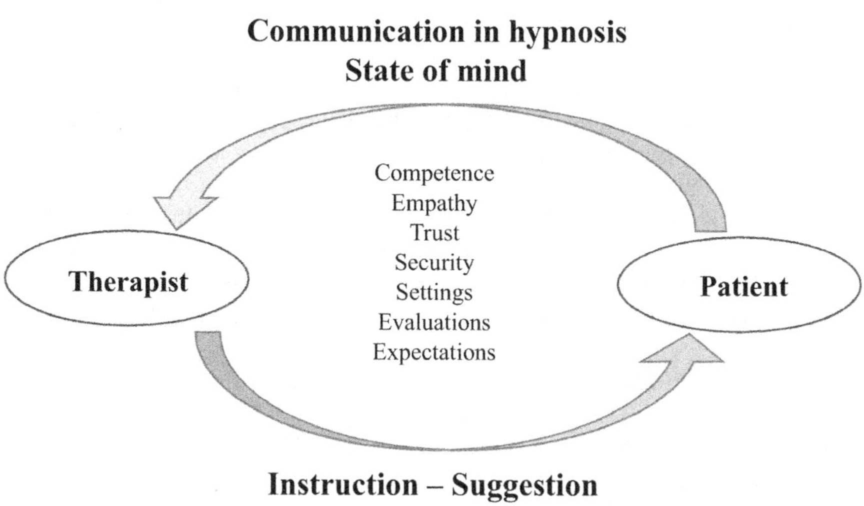

Fig. 2.3 Therapist-patient relationship

The communication between therapist and patient in hypnosis applications is referred to as *Rapport*, which is on the one hand the mutual relationship aspect between therapist and patient. On the other hand, rapport is the patient's responsiveness to the therapist's instructions and the associated certainty that the therapist verbally reaches the patient, who therefore hears him and responds appropriately. If the patient, for example, is too deeply relaxed or no longer cooperates or only follows his own thoughts or imaginations, the rapport is interrupted. The patient may then feel abandoned, follow his own negative thoughts, and the therapist then has no information about his condition. More on this in the following section.

2.5.8.1 Essential aspects of hypnotic communication

- There must be a *relationship of trust* between the therapist and the patient (Rapport).
- Hypnosis consists of the verbal and non-verbal exchange of information.
- *The therapist primarily communicates verbally.* The calmness, clarity, and directness of his statements are essential.
- *Positive and indirect formulations* (e.g., for amnesia of the number 5: "The number 5 will become irrelevant to you.")
- *Avoid:* subjunctive, nested sentences, complicated grammar, foreign words etc. Use short precise sentences; clarity in understanding is more important than high linguistic art, which confuses more in hypnosis, is hardly understood or misinterpreted. Simple sentences with word repetitions are more understandable.
- *Communicate as resource-oriented as possible,* less deficit-oriented (see Sect. 8.1.2).
- *Non-verbal information from the therapist includes:* speaking pace (slow = calming and understandable), breathing rate (slow = calm), voice pitch (low = relaxed) (e.g., Hermer and Klinzing 2004).
- *Body language and speech dynamics:* Suggestions should suggest the accompanying (desired) reactions. Example: The suggestion "*The balloon with your problem floats higher and thus you feel increasingly relieved*" should be spoken as possibly in a radio play. Here, "higher" is particularly emphasized and "*relieved*" is also spoken with clearly audible relief, as well as "relaxed" etc. The therapist verbalizing in this way should also communicate with the corresponding gestures and facial expressions. Even if he is not seen by the patient, he communicates a lot non-verbally and gives indirect and non-verbal suggestions.
- *Non-verbal information from the patient:* Hypnosis hardly deals with the very high cognitive and intellectual parts of the patient. So far, the patient has been able to make pathological evaluations such as: "All dogs bite" or "Father problems are just a construct of psychoanalysis".

With hypnosis, there is the possibility to explore the numerous emotional, evaluative, frightening etc. parts of our remembering, experiencing and living and to derive therapeutic solutions from them. So in addition to the (cognitively controlled) verbal information, we should pay particular attention to the non-verbal information from the patient and draw our conclusions from it. Thus, the verbal and non-verbal information can diverge strongly and provide different information (see Table 2.3).

Attention
The following case examples 1 (see below) and 2 to 7 (see Chap. 3) are presented concisely, as they are intended to highlight only certain methodological approaches in anamnesis and therapy or conditions of origin (learning processes in genesis) of the problem. Detailed case presentations can be found in Chap. 12.

Case Example 1 – Compulsive Washing

Clinical Picture and Diagnosis
A young woman with a strong compulsion to wash cannot report anything about the genesis of her compulsion. During the course of the exploration, she reveals that she had separated from her boyfriend and had sexual contact with him shortly afterwards. She appears slightly restless but always verbally confident. These non-verbal communications are a signal to address whether this contact was problematic for her. She then reports that she had violated her mother's strict moral rules. She becomes restless again, blushes, blinks her eyes. These are signals to address these feelings of guilt in the following hypnosis intervention. She now realizes that she feels guilty towards her mother.

Therapy
In dialogue in hypnosis, she is suggested to decide for herself what is right for her. After the therapy session, she feels more relaxed. In the next session, she reports that she felt even more relaxed afterwards and washed less. Since compulsions are very therapy-resistant, I recommend different self-control options for her further remediation.

After a few days, she reports that she now has a clear conscience regarding her sexual contacts, that she now sees herself as a moral authority—and that she now washes at a normal frequency and intensity. Without observing these minimal non-verbal movements, I would probably not have been successful.

Follow-up
The patient remains symptom-free even after a follow-up of over 20 years. ◄

2.5.8.2 Clear and Consistent Language Communication in Hypnosis

In some hypnosis treatments depending on the therapist´s theory, the patient is given the suggestion to a problem situation (e.g., sketchily exaggerated): "*You are now ten years old, have done NN and are standing in front of your father. You look at the situation and your subconscious will tell you and let you feel what a solution can be. Trust your subconscious. I will give you as much time as you need and you will report back*". Here, the patient is left alone with an impulse for a longer period of time. What does he think, feel during this time? Is he now helpless, aggressive, clueless, depressed? Does he behave like a child back then? Has he recognized something? Has he found a solution? Or does he avoid all these burdens or fears and now imagines pleasant scenes from the past or present?

During these seconds or minutes, a lot of feelings can arise, which the patient may feel exposed to and react as before or counterproductively.

Another possibility is that the patient leaves this highly aversive situation in his imaginations to spare himself or to avoid as before without a concrete solution. Especially with fears or conflict scenes, one tends to avoidance behavior, namely to leave the scene or situation to other, more beautiful imaginations or discussions.

If the therapist allows too long pauses during hypnosis, the patient can avoid this scene/confrontation with his thoughts willingly or unwillingly and switch to other (more pleasant, non-stressful) imaginations. Through this—mostly automatically used avoidance behavior he causes a negative reinforcement of his fear problem, i.e. it gets even worse (see Sect. 6.2).

> **Attention**
> If the therapist remains silent for too long during hypnosis, the patient can become insecure, then lose control over his imagination and cognitions, followed by escalating feelings of fear (feelings of aggression etc.) and his general loss of control.

2.5.8.3 Personal Close Language Communication

The therapist, who gently and continuously encourages the patient to converse with them during hypnosis, is thus always informed about the patient's feelings, reactions, or resistance to certain instructions, suggestions, or imagined scenes. Accordingly, they can proceed further with this knowledge with suggestions, etc.

- **Again and again: Simple language.** This conversation during hypnosis should follow the VAKOG principle (see Sect. 2.5.8.2) in very simple, short sentences. This way, the patient understands the messages better and can express themselves accordingly. The patient's response in hypnosis is usually delayed, slowed down, slightly slurred (like in relaxation), in simple, sometimes fragmentary sentences, almost slightly unwilling as if they do not want to be disturbed in this imagined scene.

- **Self-efficacy, Self-attribution**: Suggestions should always be oriented in such a way that the patient experiences their solutions worked out in hypnosis (through actions or ways of experiencing) as caused by themselves. They will thus cooperate better in the future, believe more in their problem-solving abilities, and thus continue to cooperate even better. In this way, they increasingly notice their self-efficacy in solving their problems; they will attribute the imagined or realized behaviors in everyday life to their own abilities (more on this in Sect. 8.2.4).

2.5.8.4 Improving Communication with VAKOG

Learning and memory research has long confirmed that learning and retention can be optimized if as many senses as possible are involved in the learning process—and thus also in different brain areas. Accordingly, recalling these learning contents is significantly facilitated if many senses and brain areas are addressed when querying the contents. If possible, they should even be deliberately woven into the instructions.

In the field of hypnosis, its induction is facilitated by formulations such as: *"You clearly feel how your eyes are getting tired, everything is becoming unclear, like blurred…"*

In the rest scene, addressing the senses is very important *"You feel the warm sun on your skin…"* and ultimately in the therapy itself, hallucinations are particularly vivid when they are stimulated accordingly: *"You clearly feel how you as a child sit on your grandmother's lap and smell her typical scent of kitchen herbs…"*

(Halsband 2004).

As many associated sensory modalities as possible should be addressed for induction, the rest scene and specific therapy scenes.

More detailed psychophysiological explanations on VAKOG are given in Table 2.2 (Kossak 2013, p. 137 ff.).

2.5.9 Notes for Practice

The same principles of communication in hypnosis apply to both suggestion and induction.

2.5.9.1 Vividness—Proximity to Experience

There is no need for a standardized test or questionnaire to determine an individual's preferred perceptions or sensory channels. When a client is asked to describe a significant rest scene for them, they will likely verbalize their preferred sensory channels. Simultaneously, they will refresh their memories of these experiences through their description of the rest scene, thereby communicating their sensory channel preferences.

Table 2.2 VAKOG—Addressing Key Sensory Modalities

Perception Area	Sensory Channel
V—Visual Perception	Seeing
A—Auditory Perception	Hearing
K—Kinesthetic Perception	Movement, Position, Force, Direction
O—Olfactory Perception	Smelling
G—Gustatory Perception	Tasting
Depending on the patient's history and perception preference, the following sensory channels may also be used:	
t—Tactile Perception Area	Touching, Feeling
t—Temperature Perception	Thermoreception
s—Pain Sensation	Nociception
v—Vestibular Perception	Balance Sense
v—Visceral Perception	Enteroception
k—Body Sensation	Proprioception

According to practice observations, patients usually prefer the sensory channels mentioned under VAKOG. Other channels are typically less significant for them. For instance, a gymnast or ballerina is likely to prioritize kinesthetic and vestibular stimuli, while a musician responds more to auditory stimuli.

Many patients are unsure about the information that is important for the anamnesis collector. Conversely, other patients describe the rest scene very abstractly, such as "Beautiful sunset." These two patient groups require subtle suggestions through exploratory questions about the scene, such as: *"Is the warmth/ the smell/ the taste etc. beautiful for you? Can you please describe how this impression (warmth etc.) affects you? What is particularly beautiful for you?"*

2.5.9.2 Vividness, Credibility

The more vivid the suggestions are spoken, the more credible they become and are followed more spontaneously. Therefore, the therapist should imagine the suggestions while speaking—as if they were present. This involves speaking calmly and relatively monotonously, but with engagement. Specifically, this includes using gestures and acting to a certain extent. Voice actors and radio play speakers do not just read text, but act in the role of the character, appearing authentic and allowing the listener to actively participate.

Examples: Vividness

- *"The balloon floats upwards"* = Look up and raise voice.
- *"She comes towards you and spreads her arms."* = Spread arms.
- *"You look down from the high tower."* = Look down.
- *"You are calmed, relieved and breathe slower, more relaxed."* = Speak in a loose, relaxed voice and sigh. ◄

Table 2.3 Comparison of the conscious rational system with the unconscious hypnosis system (inspired by: Elkins, 2017, p. 87)

Rational System (conscious)	*Modes and functions*	Hypnosis System (unconscious)
Analytical Logic	Control, Cognition	Holistic Emotion
Process-oriented	Orientation, Goal direction	Result-oriented
Conscious evaluation, weighing of arguments	Evaluations	Emotional evaluation, gut feeling, vibrations, impressions
Construction Fact check Deduction	Problem solving Therapy	Imagination Overall situation Inspiration
Rational: Through abstract symbols, words, cognitions, facts	Influence on perception	Emotional: Through targeted imaginations, images, metaphors, narratives
Conscious Effort, Striving	Effort Expenditure	Automatically effective Without effort
	Time sequences	
Slower	Information processing	Faster
Faster	Changes	Slower
Slow, more detailed—through logic and proof	Understanding, Insight	Fast, more holistic—through experiencing, living

2.5.10 Comparison of Hypnosis and Rational System

The aforementioned aspects clarify that hypnosis, with its often unconscious emotional components, and the rational dispute differ significantly in their approaches, as they are based on different processes. Therefore, it is logical to tailor the communication in hypnosis accordingly. Specifically, this means avoiding logical disputes in hypnosis. This approach only addresses the already active defense systems and defense arguments.

Hypnosis helps to address non-rational and more emotional feelings and evaluations (see Table 2.3). The comparison in this table is presented very polarizingly to emphasize the differences of the usual problem-solving methods compared to hypnosis. Simultaneously, this table can also be seen as a comparison of classical (cognitive) behavior therapy and classical hypnosis, which seemingly oppose each other in a dichotomy. In Sect. 8.4, we will demonstrate that both therapy methods complement each other in fluid transitions and are therefore extremely effective.

References

Alladin A, Alibhai A (2007) Kognitive hypnotherapiy für depression: an experimental investigation. J Exp Clin Hypn 55(2):147–165

Andersen HC (1835) Des Kaisers neue Kleider. Droemer (1938), München

Barber TX (1958) The concept of „hypnosis". J Psychol 45:115–131

Barber TX (1969) Hypnosis. A scientific approach. Van Nostrand Reinhold, New York
Barber TX (1999) A comprehensive three-dimensional theory of hypnosis. In: Kirsch I, Capafons A, Cardena-Buelna E, Amigó S (Hrsg) Clinical hypnosis and self-regulation. American Psychological Association, Washington, S 21–48
Bergin AE und Lambert ML (1978) The evaluation of therapeutic outcome. In: Garfield SL und Bergin AE (Hrsg) Handbook of psychotherapy and behavior change: an empirical analysis, 2 Aufl., Wiley, New York, S 139–189
Bernheim H (1917) Automatisme et suggestion. Librairie Felix Alcan, Paris
Berven NL (1987) Improving evaluation in counselor training and credentialing through standardized simulations. In: Edelstein BA, Berle ES (Hrsg) Evaluation and accountability in clinical training, Plenum Press, New York, S 203–229
Braffman W, Kirsch I (1999) Imaginative suggestibility and hypnotizability: an empirical analysis. J Pers Soc Psychol 77:578–587
Braid J (1843) Neurohypnology, or the rationale of nervous sleep considered in relation with animal magnetism. J. Churchill, London
Breuer J, Freud S (1895) Studien über Hysterie. Deuticke, Leipzig
Brown D, Fromm E (1986) Hypnotherapy and hypnoanalysis. Erlbaum, Hillsdale
Capafons A, Morales C, Espejo B, Cabanas S (2006) Exploratory factor analysis and psychometric properties of Valencia scale on attitudes and belief towards hypnosis, therapists version. Psicothema 18:810–815
Cardena E, Kallio S, Terhune D, Buratti S, Loof A (2007) The effects of translation and sex on hypnotizability testing. Contemp Hypn 24(4):154–160
Chapman RA (2006) Introduction to cognitive behavior therapy and hypnosis. In: Chapman RA (Hrsg) Hypnosis in cognitive behavior therapy. Springer, New York, S 3–24
Crawford HJ (1988) Differential hemispheric involvement in waking hypnosis. Paper read at the 11th International Congress of Hypnosis and Psychosomatic Medicine, Den Haag
De Vogue JT, Sachs LB (1973) The modification of hypnotic susceptability through imitative behavior. Int J Clin Exp Hypn 21:70–77
Eliade J (1960) Yoga Unsterblichkeit und Freiheit. Rascher, Zürich
Elkins GR (2017) Hypnotic Relaxation Therapy. In Elkins GR (Ed.) Handbook of Medical and Psychological Hyonosis. Springer Publ. Comp., New York, S 83-97
Gheorghiu VA (1987) The difficulty to explain and define suggestion. Vortrag, gehalten am 8.7.1987. International Symposium on Suggestion and Suggestibility, Gießen
Gheorghiu VA (2000) Suggestion und Suggestibilität: Stiefkinder der Psychologie. Vortrag, gehalten am XV. Internationalen Kongress für Hypnose, München
Gheorghium VA (1996) Die adaptive Funktion suggestionaler Phänomene. Zum Stellenwert suggestionsbedingter Einflüsse. Hypnose und Kognition 13(1):125–146
Hagl M (2019) Studien zur Wirksamkeit von Klinischer Hypnose und Hypnotherapie im Jahr 2018. Hypnose, Zeitschrift für Hypnose und Hypnotherapie 14(1+2):189–208
Haipt A, Licht K-S, Dehnen S, Deppermann S, Fallgatter AJ, Revenstorf D, Ehlis A-C (2017) Ein psychophysiologischer Vergleich von hypnotischer Trance und Entspannung. Eine Pilotstudie. Hypnose. Zeitschrift für Hypnose und Hypnotherapie 12(1+2):115–140
Heap M (2001) The alleged dangers of stage hypnosis. Contemp Hypn 17:117–126
Heidenhain R (1880) Der sogenannte thierische Magnetismus. Physiologische Beobachtungen. Breitkopf und Härtel, Leipzig
Hermer M, Klinzing HG (2004) Nonverbale Prozesse in der Psychotherapie. Dgvt-Verlag, Tübingen
Hull CJ (1933) Hypnosis and suggestibility: an experimental approach. Appleton Century Crofts, New York
Hypnose. Zeitschrift für Hypnose und Hypnotherapie (2019). Die wissenschaftlich fundierten deutschsprachigen Hypnosegesellschaften möchten Sie informieren 14(1):232.
Chaps. E (1938) Progressive relaxation. Chicago University of Chicago Press

Jambrik Z, Sebastiani I, Picano E, Ghelarducci B, Sanarcangelo EL (2005) Hypnotic modulation of flow-mediated endothelian response to mental stress. Int J Psychophysiol 55:221–227

Kihlstrom JF (1985) Hypnosis. Annu Rev Psychol 36:385–418

Kirsch I, Capafons A, Cardena-Buelna, E, Amigó S (1999) Clinical hypnosis and self-regulation: an introduction. In: Kirsch I, Capafons, A, Cardena-Buelna E, Amigó S (Hrsg) Clinical hypnosis and self-regulation: cognitive-behavioral perspective, American Psychological Association, Washington, S 3–18

Kirsch I, Lynn SJ (1999) Hypnotic involuntariness and the automaticy of everyday life. In: Kirsch I, Capafons A, Cardena-Buelna E, Amigó S (Hrsg) Clinical hypnosis and self-regulation: cognitive-behavioral perspective, American Psychological Association, Washington, S 49–72

Kirsch I (1992) The social learning theory of hypnosis. In: Bongartz W (Hrsg) Hypnosis, 175 years after Mesmer; recent developments in theory and application, Universitätsverlag Konstanz, Konstanz, S 173–186

Kirsch I (2001) The response theory of hypnosis: Expectancy and physiology. Am J Clin Hypn 44(1):69–73

Kirsch I (2011) The altered state issue: Dead or alive? Int J Clin Exp Hypn 59(3):350–362

Kirsch I, Carene E, Derbishire S, Dienes Z, Heap M, Kallio S, Mazzoni G, Naish P, Oakley D, Potter C, Walters V, Whalley M (2011) Definition von Hypnose und Hypnotisierbarkeit und deren Bezug zur Suggestion und Suggestibilität. Hypnose. Zeitschrift für Hypnose und Hypnotherapie 6(1+2):11–21

Kirsch I, Montgomery G, Sapirstein G (1995) Hypnosis as an adjunct to cognitive-behavioral psychotherapy: a meta-analysis. J Consult Clin Psychol 63:214–220

Kossak H-C (1999) Hypnose und die Kunst des Comics—oder wie man grüne Kreise in den Augen bekommen kann. Carl-Auer-Systeme Verlag, Heidelberg

Kossak H-C (2013) Hypnose. Ein Lehrbuch für Psychotherapeuten und Ärzte, 5. überarb. Aufl., Beltz, Weinheim

Kossak H-C (2020) Hypnose. In: Petermann F, Vaitl D (Hrsg) Entspannungsverfahren, 5. Aufl., BeltzPVU, Weinheim, S 99–115

Lazarus AA (1973) „Hypnosis" as a faciliator in behavior therapy. Int J Clin Exp Hypn 6:83–89

Lynn SJ, Kirsch I., Hallquist M (2008) Social cognitive theories of hypnosis. In: Nash MR, Barnier AJ (Hrsg) The Oxford Handbook of hypnosis, Oxford University Press, New York, S 111–140

Mann T (1930) Mario und der Zauberer. S. Fischer, Berlin

Mazzoni G, Venneri A, McGeown WJ, Kirsch I (2013) Neuroimaging resolution of the altered state hypothesis. Cortex 49(2):400–410

McConkey KM, Barnier AJ (2004) High hypnotizability: unity and diversity in behaviour and experience. In: Heap M, Brown BJ, Oakley DA (Hrsg), The highly hypnotizable person: Theoretical, experimental and clinical issues. Routledge, New York, S 61–84

Mialle S (1826) Exposé parordre alphabétique des cures opérées en France par le Magnétisme animal depuis Mesmer jusqu'a nos jours. Dentru, Paris

Orsillo SM, Roemer L, Block Lerner J, Tull MT (2012) Akzeptanz, Achtsamkeit und Kognitive Verhaltenstherapie. Vergleiche, Gegensätze und die Anwendbarkeit für die Behandlung von Ängsten. In: Hayes SC, Follette VM, Linehan MM (Hrsg) Achtsamkeit und Akzeptanz. Das Erweitern der kognitiv-behavioralen Tradition, dgvt-Verlag, Tübingen, S 99–137

Pawlow IP (1923) The identity of inhibition with sleep and hypnosis. Sci Monogr 17:603–608

Rogers C, Skinner BF (1956) Some issues concerning the control of human behaviour: a symposium. Science 124:1057–1066

Schultz JH (1932) Das Autogene Training. Thieme, Leipzig-Stuttgart

Shor RE, Orne MT (1962) Harvard Group Scale of Hypnotic Suseptability, Form A. Consulting Psychologists Press. Palo Alto

Trinder H, Salkovskis PM (1994) Personally relevant intrusions outside the laboratory: long-term suppression increases intrusion. Behav Res Ther 32(8):833–842

Vaitl D (2020) Autogenes Training. In: Petermann F, Vaitl D (Hrsg), Entspannungsverfahren. Ein Praxishandbuch, 4. Aufl., Beltz, Weinheim, S 62–80

Vogt O (1895a) Zur Kenntnis des Wesens und der psychologischen Bedeutung des Hypnotismus. Zeitschrift für Hypnotismus 3:277–340

Vogt O (1895b) Zur Kenntnis des Wesens und der psychologischen Bedeutung des Hypnotismus. Zeitschrift für Hypnotismus 5(32):122–229

Wegner DM, Schneider DJ, Carter S, White T (1987) Paradoxical effects of thought suppression. J Pers Soc Psychol 53:5–13

Weitzenhoffer AM, Hilgard ER (1958) Stanford Hypnotic susceptability scale, forms A and B. Consulting Psychologists Press, Palo Alto

Weitzenhoffer AM (1989) Betrachtungen der Hypnotisierbarkeit. Mehr als dreißig Jahre später. Experimentelle und klinische Hypnose 5(1):63–73

Whitehead S, Noller P, Sheehan PW (2008) The hypnotist in the hypnosis interaction: the impact of first impression on perceptions of hypnotisability. Int J Clin Exp Hypn 56(4):394–424

Wickramasekera I (1971) Effects of "hypnosis" and task motivational instructions in attempting to influence the "voluntary" self-deprivation of money. J Pers Soc Psychol 19:311–314

Wolberg LR (1982) Hypnosis: is it for you? Dembner Books, New York

Woody E, Sattler P (2017) Hypnotizability. In: Elkins GR (Hrsg) Handbook of Medical and Psychological Hypnosis, Springer, New York, S 35–41

Neuropsychology of Hypnosis

3

Contents

Numerous research groups from various schools of thought have confirmed that, for instance, a hypnotic trance induction triggers plastic changes in the human brain (e.g., Rainville et al. 2002; Spiegel and Kosslyn 2004; Halsband and Hinterberger 2010). The numerous effects of hypnosis, often referred to as mysterious by laypeople, can now also be explained neuropsychologically. The comprehensive results from the specialist literature can only be presented here in small sample excerpts.

H.-C. Kossak, *Cognitive-behavioral Psychotherapy for Anxiety*, https://doi.org/10.1007/978-3-662-69099-4_3

3.1 Induction—Introduction to Hypnosis

The effect of the hypnosis introduction is determined by the client's expectations to behave as they believe one should behave under hypnosis. This includes the traditional assumption that being hypnotized involves sleep, fatigue, and closing one's eyes.

Accordingly, instructions or suggestions are given to become increasingly tired, then to close the eyes and continue to relax. The therapist uses their knowledge that the instruction to fixate a point for a long time leads to eye fatigue, associated with dryness, redness of the sclera, and burning eyes. They can observe this process precisely and describe it to the patient as a suggestion. As a result, the patient assumes that the therapist is causing these changes through their suggestions. Continuous feedback (= differential reinforcement) then leads to eye closure and relaxation, associated with the subsequent concentration on breathing.

Neuropsychological Brain Changes

Since the inception of the scientific investigations of hypnosis and its effective factors, researchers have been searching for their neurophysiological substrates, i.e., specific brain areas, their activities, functions, and cooperations.

The therapist's monotonous speech, rhythmic noises (metronome), or rhythmic eye movements (by pendulum) cause a synchronization of the reticular formation with the cortex (Gellhorn and Loofbourrow 1963). Upon eye closure, there is then an increasing parietal and occipital, and then frontal alpha wave activity.

Hypnosis is closely associated with power in the theta band and changes in gamma activities. This oscillation likely plays a significant role in the recording and memory in the declarative memory and emotionally in the limbic system (Jensen et al. 2015).

The hypnotizability measured in the test takes the form of a normal distribution curve (Woody and Banier 2008). The EEG phase synchronization likely even indicates the degree of hypnotizability (Bagdadi and Nasrabadi 2012).

In hypnosis, the theta band activity in the EEG is increased in highly hypnotizable individuals, which suggests their higher focused attention (Graffin et al. 1995). The hypnosis induction likely causes a qualitative change in the organization of special control systems in the brain of the highly hypnotizable individuals (Jamieson and Burgess 2014). Depending on the tasks set, different cortical and subcortical processes are activated in hypnosis; however, the brain of the highly hypnotizable individuals in hypnosis performs similarly to other brains, but better (Crawford 2001).

Overall, hypnosis can be seen as a guided introduction to various states of self-perception, consciousness, or cognition (Hinterberger et al. 2011).

3.2 Hypnosis as a Relaxation Method

Neuropsychological data clearly indicate that hypnosis, particularly in highly hypnotizable individuals, induces strong relaxation effects. This is why the restful scene created by hypnosis, such as "Green Meadow", depending on the client, situation, and symptomatology, induces deep relaxation (see below). Conversely, for those with low hypnotizability, hypnosis does not significantly differ from other relaxation methods in terms of relevant physiological measurements.

Relaxation methods are particularly beneficial in the treatment of fears as they lead to a general calming, especially of the amygdala's alarm system. This helps to provide the patient with increasing security and to tolerate and endure confrontation with the real or imagined content of fear. Since the patient maintains verbal contact with the therapist, they can trust that the therapist will not lead them into an overly threatening situation and then abandon them (Elkins 2017).

3.2.1 Hypnotizability and Relaxation

In highly suggestible individuals, the level of wakefulness decreases compared to relaxation, and their heart rate variability also decreases. During trance, the proportions of high frequencies in the total heart rate decrease, suggesting a reduced parasympathetic influence during trance (Haipt et al. 2017). Highly hypnotizable individuals exhibit higher alpha activity in hypnosis, indicating a highly relaxed state of wakefulness (e.g., Williams and Gruzelier 2001), as does their high theta power (Konrad et al. 2004).

Hypnotic responsiveness is stable, suggesting that genetic factors may play a role. Highly hypnotizable individuals have a larger rostrum, an area in the corpus callosum (Horton et al. 2004). Their speed of information processing suggests a faster neural network. Their improved dopaminergic state indicates a more effective anterior frontal executive control system and higher supervisory attention (Crawford et al. 2004).

3.2.2 Application of Relaxation Techniques

Traditional relaxation methods such as autogenic training or progressive muscle relaxation achieve the desired relaxation, but require a relatively long practice time of about 6–8 sessions until patients feel deeply relaxed and can initiate and maintain relaxation on their own. In the everyday practice of psychotherapists or doctors, this can be a hindrance, as often time is pressing until healing, for example, in time-bound problems such as exam fears, job interviews, public appearances. It is not always possible to provide relaxation instruction at the required time or to schedule it at short notice. Participation in various groups is useful, but rarely will a group therapy place for relaxation training be available at the desired time in one's own or a friend's practice.

Advantage of Hypnosis Relaxation: Time Economy
Hypnosis relaxation offers the significant advantage of being quickly effective. In my practice experience spanning over five decades, almost all patients have immediately responded with relaxation to the rest scene of their choice. After the first application, in which the rest scene including induction took about 10 minutes, they usually feel deeply relaxed, comfortable, and satisfied. This time economy is of great value in cases of very strong anxieties or when treatment is needed promptly.

I can report only one exception; here the client had strong fears of losing control, even though there was great trust in the therapist. Even a relaxation CD did not help. His profession as an internal auditor in a large company may have contributed to this attitude.

3.3 Activation of Relevant Neurophysiological Systems in Hypnosis

Hypnosis can generate various hallucinations, which target specific networks and, for example, alleviate pain. They influence histamine production in the skin, the immune system, peripheral circulation, blood coagulation, and temperature regulation, among others. These changes are necessary for healing in numerous diseases that respond to appropriate suggestions. In these suggestions, the therapist utilises the patient's previous learning experiences.

Example: Heat and Cold Suggestions

Since each of us has experienced the warmth of a fireplace or stove and the cold of a frozen windowpane with our hands, these dermal experiences of temperature, comfort, and coziness have been stored in our brain in the relevant networks. When re-experiencing fewer of these accompanying conditions, the organism can draw on these memories. The same can be achieved by intensely looking at, for example, holiday photos, as this stimulates memories of the holiday experiences, evoking the accompanying perceptions and moods. ◄

VAKOG
Good suggestions utilise the client's stored experiences by addressing these experiences directly through vivid formulations and the use of VAKOG (see Table 2.2). In doing so, they activate the corresponding networks of physical and emotional experiences.

Such suggestions then trigger, for example, the vasodilation of the blood vessels in the hand through a fireplace suggestion. With the suggestion to touch the frost flowers on the windowpane with the palm of the hand, the hand will react with vasoconstriction according to its neuronal engrams. Both are each objectively and significantly measurable in their effects.

The unprepared suggestion without context: "Your hand is getting warm" will therefore hardly have any influence on the circulation. But the suggestion "You are sitting by the campfire/fireplace and stretch your hands towards the pleasant warmth of the fire and clearly feel this pleasant warmth on your palms .... etc." will be successful after a short time.

Effect on Central Control and Filter Systems

The numerous neurological findings collected in recent years increasingly provide differentiated hypotheses about the work of certain brain areas and their connections in one, usually several, networks. With this basic knowledge, the effect of certain suggestions becomes more recognisable at the neuronal level.

While it was previously assumed that, for example, suggestions for pain reduction work directly on the affected organ, it has been proven that hypnosis suggestions are effective centrally in the brain in the responsible pain center.

Central Effect of the Suggestions

The suggestions directed at a system such as pain work through specific control mechanisms at the main pain centers. This top-down effect of suggestions in hypnosis can also be observed in numerous other suggestions. This addresses central filter and control processes that objectively show their effects (e.g., Spiegel and Spiegel, 2004; Mirror and Mirror 1987; Kosslyn et al. 2001; Landry and Raz 2017).

3.4 Can Hypnosis Influence Cognitive Factors?

With these neurologically central effects of hypnosis, the question arises to what extent hypnosis can also influence cognitive factors.

3.4.1 Simulation

Ultimately, hypnosis with its possibly externally visible signs can be simulated in such a way that it cannot be distinguished from real or simulated behaviours by experts, nor their depth.

Often therapists name slowed speech, slowed motor skills, reduced facial expressions with deep relaxation of the facial muscles as typical signs of hypnosis. However, all of this does not have to be true if the patient is dealing with a highly stressful experience in hypnosis and is afraid or angry.

So for safety, it only helps to refer to the patient's statements in dialogue during hypnosis—and to rely on these corresponding to the patient's subjective and objective reality.

3.4.2 The Concept of Truth

It has become clear that we encounter the problem of truth in the context of hypnosis:

- Therapist and patient may hold different personal "truths".
- The subjective truth in hypnosis can differ from the objective one.
- In the context of hypnosis, the patient can behave in a manner that is appropriate for them.
- Is there an objective truth in psychotherapy?
- Is there a definition of normality against which truth can be judged?
- Truth has an ethical-moral basis, not an objective one (Stavemann 2014).

Credibility—Simulation—Reality in Hypnosis

- Statements made in hypnosis do not necessarily correspond to reality.
- Statements made in hypnosis can be simulated, confabulated, and contaminated by other experiential and memory contents, i.e., altered.
- In psychotherapy, suffering is sometimes caused by the subjective reality, such as being affected or damaged in a certain way by a specific person or situation.
- Sometimes, it is sufficient to therapeutically change this subjective reality, for example, through reframing (see Sect. 8.3.4).
- Sometimes, it also needs to be clarified whether the problem at hand has actually occurred in the form experienced and presented by the patient.

> **Important**
> As a proven correct conclusion of the aforementioned presentations, it is considered:
>
> Statements obtained in hypnosis that can lead to serious burdens on other people—such as in cases of suspected abuse or other criminal acts—cannot be considered objective. They serve only for hypothesis formation and must always be corroborated by objective findings, statements, evidence, etc.

3.4.3 Free Will, External Influence, and Criminal Acts in Hypnosis

Properly conducted psychotherapy will always proceed in a client-centered manner and take into account the wishes and boundaries of the patient. However, this can also lead to critical situations in which the patient has to confront their anxiety situation. This may seem against their will at the moment, but it is in line with the therapy contract agreed upon. The therapist will certainly respect existing psychological, physical, and moral boundaries.

With the reduced critical ability of the patient in hypnosis, they can experience their self-generated actions as externally controlled. They may perceive this as intrusive and complain about it in case of insufficient preparation or unfavorable constellation. The neuropsychological findings on this are detailed in Sect. 3.4.4.

Criminal Acts in Hypnosis

There are indeed cases where lay hypnotists took advantage of their client's social situation or suggested other environmental conditions in hypnosis (e.g., hot summer requires taking off clothes). These missteps clearly represent the abuse of hypnosis and the client. However, this is not typical or unique to hypnosis, but can occur in many close relationships such as therapy (Orne 1983). People in hypnosis do not lose control over their behavior when the treatment is correctly performed (American Psychological Association 1994). Thus, they cannot be induced to commit criminal acts in hypnosis, even if crime novels and films suggest it.

3.4.4 Hypnosis and the Influence of Will—Subjectively Experienced or Objectively Present?

A question and associated fear that has arisen since the inception of hypnosis is that of the influence of will and the loss of reality during hypnosis.

- When there is a strong focus on a stimulus, attention is directed solely towards it. In this process, the brain selectively pays attention to the stimuli in such a way that other stimuli are either not consciously perceived or barely noticed alongside these particularly emphasized stimuli (Simons and Chabris 1999).
- The belief in the reality of what is experienced during hypnosis depends on the strength of hypnotizability, that is, the ability to be strongly absorbed by inner experiences (Sutcliffe et al. 1979).
- The aforementioned filter and control processes created in hypnosis objectively interfere with perceptions, such as pain.
- In voluntary actions, the activation of the responsible prefrontal Cortex occurs (Crawford 1996, see above). Hypnosis reduces the connection between the dorsolateral Cortex and the anterior cingulum, resulting in reduced critical ability (Nordby et al. 1999; Gruzelier 1998), which is reflected in the restriction of verbal fluency and reduced error detection.
- Identical active movements are processed differently by the brain in the parietal Cortex and in the cerebellum, depending on whether they are evaluated as self-caused or caused by an external force. Hypnotic suggestions lead to overactivity of the cerebellar-parietal network; this then causes self-generated actions to be experienced as externally caused (Blakemore et al. 2003).

> **Important**
> Hypnosis influences numerous brain activities, which are then experienced as externally controlled, even though they were initiated by suggestions from the subject themselves (Kirsch 2011).

3.4.5 Hypnosis and Perception Influence—Reality of Inner Images

Numerous experiments show that inner images are as real for the brain as objectively seen images. The MRI results clarify this: real objects seen activate certain areas in the brain, which are identical to the brain activities that occur when this object is only imagined (Kosslyn et al. 2000). This means, on the one hand, the brain cannot distinguish between real "experienced" and "merely imagined". Thus, the small colourful pixels that make up a television image are also experienced as real. They trigger the intended emotions such as hate, love, longing, similar to the real situation.

> **Important**
> The person in hypnosis experiences themselves as subjectively real in the scene suggested to them, for example, the rest scene or in their therapy scene, given sufficient cooperation and hypnotizability.

3.4.6 Hypnosis and Reality

> **Neuropsychological Effects:**
> Hypnosis and perception of reality (according to Spiegel and Kosslyn 2004):
>
> - Intense focus on internally generated mental images.
> - Expectations are generated during perception processing, which in turn influence perception. This leads, among other things, to stable illusions.
> - Hypnosis instructions (suggestions) to change perception lead to corresponding changes in the relevant cortices. This makes the perceived change feel real.
> - Due to the specific processing in hypnosis, people react to the words of the suggestion and manipulate their perception accordingly. Without hypnosis, people react to perception as reality and then manipulate the words.

> **Important**
> Hypnosis creates reality in the brain (Peter 2008).

3.5 Creating the Rest Scene

These scientifically based knowledge about physiology must be utilised in the development of the relaxations scene. If the patient is merely asked what kind of rest scene they desire, they may be at a loss, as they can associate little with the term spontaneously. However, if it is vividly and concretely explained that a pleasantly relaxing imaginative scene will be needed later, such as a beautiful holiday experience where the patient has ample time and enjoys the tranquillity, then this scene could be a holiday memory of a beautiful beach, a pleasant landscape, a forest walk, or a beautiful meadow. This provides the patient with a model of what will be needed next and can relatively quickly offer them a pleasant scene. The patient should describe this as vividly as possible—with VAKOG support from the therapist. Careful observation of their facial expressions often reveals which impressions are pleasant and should be used for the rest scene.

Example: Individual Design of the Rest Scene

If the patient opts for the "standard scene", one cannot assume that both patient and therapist share the same relaxation ideas about the beach. Therefore, one should inquire about the "beach": in which country, steep coast or flat sand, season, typical plants, noises, windy or calm, etc.

During this vivid conversation, the patient develops more and more memories of the associated beautiful, relaxing impressions. The therapist receives more and more information, which they will then use as suggestions of warmth, peace, relaxation etc. Through the exploration of the rest scene, the patient becomes increasingly relaxed, so that the suggestions for the rest scene following the induction become effective quite quickly. ◄

3.6 The Posthypnotic Task

This term posthypnotic task encompasses an instruction or suggestion given during hypnosis to behave, feel, or remember in a certain way after hypnosis at a specific time or on a defined occasion. The posthypnotic task with its effects is considered typical for hypnotic behaviour and is therefore an item in the SHSS: A (see Sect. 2.5.2.1).

Scholz et al. (2008, p. 117) critically note: "A posthypnotic task is not a command in the sense of a request or even an order, because with the consent to clinical hypnosis, the patient expressly agrees that the hypnotherapist focuses on the implicit, i.e., automatically running (unconscious) information processing processes of the patient."

Sometimes, test subjects behave like automatons when performing their task, but only if they assume that this is part of "hypnotic" behaviour (Spanos et al. 1987). Since the posthypnotic task is performed automatically, i.e., without the conscious cooperation of the patient, both the explicit and the implicit memory are addressed (Scholz et al. 2008). Overall, the effects of the posthypnotic task are effects of expectations and social and cognitive conditions. The duration of the effect depends on many factors, including suggestibility (Berrigan et al. 1991).

In the clinical area, posthypnotic suggestions are used, for example, for pain reduction, compliance with prescribed medication intake, anxiety reduction in the relevant situation, temptation situation in food control, diet adherence and smoking cessation. In the case of exam and performance anxiety, they reduce excitement, fear and worry at the required time of the exam (Scholz 2009). The experimentally tested period between task assignment and its execution can last up to several months.

Neuropsychological explanations for this are still very rare. It is clear that instructions are given to the hippocampus (working memory, short-term memory) and the prefrontal cortex (long-term memory) (see Sect. 5.1). My assumption is that with precise formulation of the triggers and goals of the relevant remembering, the same processes take place as with concentrated learning.

Design of the Formulations for the Posthypnotic Task (Scholz et al. 2008; Barnier and McConkey 1996)

- Compatibility with the person's attitudes and beliefs
- Action-oriented formulations work better than receptive ones
- Use of an existing motivation for change
- Positive formulations
- Short, concise formulations
- Concrete formulations

Scholz (2013) uses a formulation algorithm for the posthypnotic task, which we will largely follow or modify slightly in therapy (see Sect. 11.16).

To build self-confidence, autonomy, self-efficacy, and self-control, for example, in controlling fear behavior, the posthypnotic suggestion precisely defines under which stimulus conditions (e.g., seeing a dog) cognitive self-control should occur (see Fig. 3.1).

3.7 Aspects of the Instruction of the Posthypnotic Task

- The instruction for the execution of the relevant (emotional, motor, etc.) posthypnotic behavior must be clearly linked to a *trigger stimulus*.
- The trigger stimuli used for posthypnotic tasks should be formulated very precisely and differentiated, as well as the behavior to follow.
- *External stimulus conditions* for triggering posthypnotic behavior are: seeing, hearing, feeling certain stimuli in phobics such as a dog, boss, high building, injection needle.

The initial stimulus and its consequences ⟹

Stimulus	**S1 -**	**S2 - R1**	**S3 - R2**	**S4 - R3**	**S5**	**R4**
Definition	Remembering activity	Time when?	Place Where?	Action Which one?	Execution When?	required. action?
Order: Borrow book NN		Search Monday	office at the desk.	Put the book in your pocket.	next Day See A.	Give book

Fig. 3.1 Posthypnotic task: Stimulus definition and discrimination
The posthypnotic order precisely defines the instructions for the triggers and their reactions in the action chain. The individual actions are in turn triggering stimuli for the next behavior in the chain. As with all more complex orders, the subgoals are also precisely defined. "If … then."
The instruction here is: "*Please lend me the book NN. When you are in the office on Monday, please look for the book when you are at your desk. Then put the book in your briefcase. When you see me the next day, you will give me the book.*"Note on these and the following graphic representations of operant behaviors:
An attempt was made to realize a simple and clear representation of the sometimes complex behavior sequences. This should not lead to classifying behavior therapy as reductionist and seeing behavior solely as pure stimulus-response sequences.

- *Internal stimuli:*
  - Cognitive stimuli (= thoughts) such as: "*Whenever you think of NN.*"
  - Emotional stimuli: "*When you feel the emotion NN, then...*"
  - Physiological stimuli: "*When you feel this tension in your body, then...*"
- Thus, almost any stimuli can trigger certain behaviors and thus also serve as triggers for the posthypnotic task.
- Ultimately, *time specifications* can also be used as triggers "*Next Wednesday, when NN occurs, then...*"

References

American Psychological Association (APA) (1994) Statement on memories of sexual abuse. Int J Clin Exp Hypn 42(4):261–264

Baghdadi G, Nasrabadi AM (2012) EEG phase synchronization during hypnosis induction. J Med Eng Tech 36(4):222–229

Barnier AJ, McConkey KM (1996) Action and desire in posthypnotic responding. Int J Clin Exp Hyp 44(2):120–139

Berrigan LP, Kurtz RM, Stabile J und Strube (1991) Durability of „posthypnotic suggestions" as a function of type of trance depth. Int J Clin Exp Hypn 39(1): 24–38

Blakemore S-J, Oakley DA, Frith CD (2003) Delusion of alien control in the normal brain. Neuropsychologica 41:1058–1067

Crawford H (1996) Cerebral brain dynamics of mental imagery: evidence and issues for hypnosis. In Kunzendorf RG, Spanos NP, Sheikh AA (Hrsg) Hypnosis and imagination. Baywood, Amityville, S 253–282

Crawford HN (2001) Neuropsychophysiology of hypnosis: Towards an understanding of how hypnotic interventions work. Wiley, New York

Crawford HJ, Horton E, Lichtenberg P (2004) Die Neurobiologie der Hypnose Wie beeinflussen Gene, Neuroanatomie sowie Faktoren der Informationsgeschwindigkeitsprozesse die hypnotische Antwortbereitschaft? Hypnose und Kognition 21(1):93–116

Elkins GR (2017) Hypnotic relaxation therapy. In: Elkins GR (Hrsg) Handbook of medical and psychological hypnosis. Springer, New York, S 83–97

Gellhorn E, Loofbourrow GN (1963) Emotions and emotional disorders. Harper and Row, New York

Graffin NF, Ray WJ, Lundy R (1995) EEG concomitants of hypnosis and hypnotic susceptability. J Abnorm Psychol 104(1):123–131

Gruzelier JH (1998) A working model of the neurophysiology of hypnosis: a review of the evidence. Contemp Hypn 15:3–21

Haipt A, Licht K-S, Dehnen S, Deppermann S, Fallgatter AJ, Revenstorf D, Ehlis A-C (2017) Ein psychophysiologischer Vergleich von hypnotischer Trance und Entspannung. Eine Pilotstudie. Hypnose. Zeitschrift für Hypnose und Hypnotherapie 12(1+2):115–140

Halsband U, Hinterberger T (2010) Veränderungen der Plastizität im Gehirn unter Hypnose. Hypnose. Zeitschrift für Hypnose und Hypnotherapie 5(1+2):33–50

Hinterberger T, Schoner J, Halband U (2011) Analsis of electroencephalogical state patterns and changes during hypnosis induction. Int J Clin Exp Hypn 59(2):165–179

Horton JE, Crawford HJ, Harrington G, Drowns JH (2004) Increased anterior corpus callosum size assoziated positively with hypnotizability and the ability to control pain. Brain 127:1741–1747

Jamieson GA, Burgess AP (2014) Hypnotic induction is followed by state-like changes in the organization of EEG functional connectivity in the theta and beta frequencecy bands in high-hypnotically susceptible individuals. Front Hum Neurosci 24(8):528

Jensen MP, Tomoroni A, Hakimian S (2015) Brain oscillations, hypnosis and hypnotizability. Am J Clin Hypn 57(3):230–325

Kirsch I (2011) The altered state issue: dead or alive? Int J Clin Exp Hypn 59(3):350–362

Konrad B, Deeb S, Scholz OB (2004) Motorische Imagination in Hypnose. Alpha- und Thetapower während motorischer Imagination in Hypnose. Hypnose und Kognition 21(1+2):183–203

Kosslyn SM, Ganis G, Thompson WL (2001) Neural foundations of imagery. Nat Rev Neurosci 2:635–642

Kosslyn SM, Thompson WL, Constantini-Ferrando MF, Alpert NM, Spiegel D (2000) Hypnotic visual illusion alters color processing in the brain. Am J Psychiatry 157(8):1279–1284

Landry M, Raz A (2017) Neuropsychology of hypnosis. In Elkins GR (Hrsg) Handbook of Medical and Psychological Hypnosis. Springer Publ Comp, New York, S 19–28

Nordby H, Hugdahl K, Jasiukaitis P, Spiegel D (1999) Effects of hypnotizability on performance of a Stroop task and event-related potentials. Percept Mot Skills 88(3 Pt 1):819–830

Orne MT (1983) Kann man unter Hypnose jemanden zwingen, etwas zu tun, was er sonst nicht tun würde. Experimentelle und klinische Hypnose 1(1):19–33

Peter B (2008) Wie Hypnose im Gehirn Wirklichkeit schafft. Hypnose. Zeitschrift für Hypnose und Hypnotherapie 3(1+2):127–148

Rainville P, Hofbauer RK, Bushnell MC, Duncan GH, Pricem DD (2002) Hypnosis modulates activity in brain structurse involved in the regulation of consciousness. J Cogn Neurosci 14(6):887–901

Scholz OB (2013) Hypnotherapie bei chronischen Schmerzerkrankungen. 2. überarb. Aufl., Huber, Bern

Scholz OB, Bleek B, Schlien A (2008) Suggestionen, die erst nach der Hypnose wirken sollen: Präsentation einer Posthypnose-Aufgabe. Zeitschrift für Hypnose und Hypnotherapie 3(1+2):117–126

Scholz OB (2009) Was erinnern Personen mit Prüfungs- und Leistungsangst von einer Posthypnotischen Aufgabe (PHA)? Deutsche Zeitschrift für Zahnärztliche Hypnose 15(1):29–50

Simons DJ, Chabris CF (1999) Gorillas in our midst: sustained inattentional blindness for dynamic events. Perception 28:1059–1074

Spanos NP, Menary E, Brett PJ, Gross W, Ahmed Q (1987) Failure of posthypnotic responding to occur outside the experimental setting. J Abnorm Psychol 96(1):52–57

Spiegel D, Kosslyn S (2004) Glauben ist sehen: Die Neuropsychologie der Hypnose. Hypnose. Zeitschrift für Hypnose und Hypnotherapie 21(1+2):119–137

Spiegel H, Spiegel D (2004) Trance and treatment. Clinical uses of hypnosis Arlington, 2 Aufl., American Psychiatric Publishing, VA

Stavemann HH (2014) KVT-Praxis. Strategien und Leitfäden für die Integrative KVT. Beltz, Weinheim

Sutcliffe JP, Perry CW, Shehan PW (1979) Relation of some aspects of imagery and fantasy to hypnotic susceptibility. J Abnorm Psychol 76:279–287

Williams JD, Gruzelier JH (2001) Differentiation of hypnosis and relaxation by analysis of narrow band theta and alpha frequencies. Int J Clin Exp Hyp 49(3):185–206

Woody ET, Barnier AJ (2008) Hypnosis scales for the 21st century: what do we need and how should we use them? In: Nash MR, Barnier AJ (Hrsg) Oxford handbook of hypnosis; theory, research and practice. Oxford University Press, Oxford, S 255–282

Anxiety

4

Contents

Intensive research has been conducted on the fundamental feeling of fear, as it is a significant aspect in the existence of almost all higher living beings.

H.-C. Kossak, *Cognitive-behavioral Psychotherapy for Anxiety*,
https://doi.org/10.1007/978-3-662-69099-4_4

4.1 The Function of Anxiety

In evolution, anxiety is particularly significant, as it is a mechanism for the protection and survival of the individual and the species. In real or perceived situations, anxiety functions to heighten vigilance and activate increased physical strength to either escape the dangerous situation or to stand up for defence, i.e., *Fight-or-Flight* (Warwitz 2016). To ensure a high survival rate in evolutionary history, individuals react relatively quickly, possibly even to minimal threats (Nesse 2001). This can easily trigger false alarms.

Much has been published, experimented, and numerous theories have been proposed about anxiety in philosophy, psychology, and physiology. The specific discussion about this will not be addressed here. Instead, we primarily want to address the aspects relevant to our method.

4.2 Clinical Classification of Anxiety Disorders

Assuming knowledge of diagnostics according to the ICD-10-GM-2020, a brief summary of the anxiety disorders relevant to us follows (see Table 4.1).

The following information is also taken from the ICD-10 (2020).

Epidemiology:
Anxiety disorders are among the most common mental illnesses (Kessler et al. 2005a, b). The lifetime prevalence is internationally at 14% to 29%, and in Germany, it is at 15% (Jacobi et al. 2014).

Differential Diagnoses—Examples (ICD-10):

- Organic anxiety disorders (F06.4)
- Substance-related disorders (F1)
- Schizophrenia (F20)
- Seizure disorders
- Anxiety symptoms that can occur as part of physical disease or disorder states such as: Hyperthyroidism, hypoglycemic states, pheochromocytoma, seizure disorders, cardiovascular diseases.

Table 4.1 Classification of anxiety disorders according to ICD-10-GM-2020

F40. Phobic disorders	F41. Other anxiety disorders
F40.0 Agoraphobia	F41.0 Panic disorders (episodic paroxysmal anxiety)
F40.00 Without indication of a panic disorder	F41.1 Generalized anxiety disorder
F40.01 With panic disorder	F41.2 Anxiety and depressive disorder, mixed
F40.1 Social phobia	F41.3 Other mixed anxiety disorders
F40.2 Specific (isolated) phobia	F41.8 Other specific anxiety disorders
F40.8 Other phobic disorders	F41.9 Anxiety disorders; not further specified
F40.9 Phobic disorder, not further specified	

Comorbidity:
There is an increased risk of also suffering from other anxiety disorders, depression, somatoform disorders, addiction problems, and personality disorders (Flick et al. 1993).

Therapy:
The focus is on a multimodal therapy concept, which prioritizes cognitive behavioral therapy, followed by pharmacotherapy and psychodynamic psychotherapy (Kessler et al. 2005a, b).

4.3 Components of Anxiety

Fear is multidimensional, as it manifests in various forms and affects different components of the organism. The following will briefly outline these, as far as possible.

Numerous theories exist, based on very different theoretical directions, especially regarding the origin, description, maintenance, and therapy of fear. Since our primary focus is on therapy, particularly the practical application of a combination of hypnosis and behaviour therapy, we will not delve into complex theoretical discussions here. Instead, we will focus on the essential models in behaviour theory.

4.3.1 Early Anxiety Models

In the early stages of scientific research, it was assumed that fear was determined by three factors.

The Three-Component Model—e.g. by Lang (1968)

- Physiology = Rapid heartbeat, sweating, shortness of breath etc.
- Behaviour = Escape and avoidance (motor skills)
- Cognition = Narrowing of perception and thinking—especially on stimuli relevant for dangers

In this definition, only escape and avoidance are defined as behaviour, that is, motor-visible and recordable behaviour. This corresponds to the then view that only directly and objectively detectable and recordable reactions were considered (open) behaviour.

> **Note**
> With the expansion of the early and orthodox views of behaviour theory, it was recognised that beyond these visible behaviours, emotions, imaginations, and cognitions are also to be described as (covert) behaviour, even if they are only subjective and not directly detectable.

4.3.1.1 The New Component: Cognitions

In the further development of behaviour theory, it was recognised that non-visible behaviour (covert behaviour) is also effective. This includes cognitions with their attributions, motivation, and imagination.

4.3.1.2 Brief Definition of Cognitions

- Mental processes such as thoughts, judgments, opinions, attitudes, intentions.
- Information processing processes: Learning, knowledge processing, thinking, problem-solving.
- Cognitions are what one thinks about oneself, the social and physical environment—in relation to their past, present, and future.

4.3.1.3 The Evolution of Cognitive Theories

Research branches such as motivation research and attribution research have developed accordingly. This situates us directly in the field of cognitive-behavioural causation of disorders and their therapy, which are elaborated in Sect. 6.1.4.

4.3.1.3.1 The Influence of Cognitions and Emotions on Each Other

Emotional disorders can arise and be maintained by cognitive disorders (Beck 1963, 1967; Ellis 1994; Wells 2011), that is, by a dysfunction in information processing. These dysfunctions cause assumptions and beliefs, such as self-deprecation, inability, and automatic thoughts. Their focus in control processing is emphasized by Meichenbaum (1985/2003) (see Sect. 6.1.4).

4.3.1.3.2 Irrational Thoughts and Schemas

In anxiety disorders, there is an *overestimation* of danger, which generates emotional arousal. This arousal, in a recurring feedback loop, is interpreted as confirmation of the fear. This is often associated with danger and further negative events are "derived" (i.e., irrational thoughts). Eventually, complex cognitive *"schemas"* emerge, such as being incapable, unloved, rejected, or *generalizations* like "always, none, never," where distinctions are required. These then lead to *general negative beliefs* about oneself and then, for example, to social withdrawal.

4.3.1.3.3 Cognitive Distortions and Safeguarding

If danger is only suspected in small amounts in anxiety patients, the "danger schema" is activated, which causes distortions (i.e., biases) in information processing and then initiates precautions such as the typical safeguarding behaviour (Salkovskis 1991), which in turn maintains the anxious behaviour. This is then accompanied by the physiological and motor behaviours characteristic of anxiety.

4.3.1.3.4 Negative Automatic Thoughts

Also essential are the mostly uncontrollablenegative automatic thoughts (NATs) and ruminations, which impose themselves in verbal and pictorial form

(= Imaginations) (Borkovec et al. 1983). Attempts to suppress or control these almost compulsive thoughts paradoxically intensify them. They are thereby placed in the focus of attention and are given even more attention. Here, identical mechanisms are effective as with negative suggestions (compare Sect. 2.5.1.2).

4.3.1.3.5 Detailed Analysis of Behaviour

A finer distinction of behavioural components helps to view mental processes, diseases, symptoms—primarily anxiety—in a much more differentiated way. This variety of possible components is overlooked according to the old three-component models. To give special consideration to the numerous cognitive factors of behaviour, especially anxious behaviour, I have tried to develop a manageable system (Kossak 1989). From this, the individual aspects of diagnosis can be more easily recognized and therapy plans can be derived.

Here, only the Anxieties ICD-10 F40x and F41x are referred to.

4.3.2 The Model of the Seven-Behaviour-Components of Anxiety

The three-component model of anxiety was revised by me (1989) for practical considerations and is here expanded to seven components.

The Components

Compared to the previously used three components, the following changes or extensions have been made:

- New: Inclusion of *emotions* as important control and regulatory elements of behaviour.
- New: Inclusion of *imaginations* as orientation and regulatory elements of behaviour.
- New: Division of cognition into its operational components: *cognitions* (thoughts), *attributions* (evaluations) and *motivation* (expectations, goals).
- Retention of: *motor skills* and *physiology.*

Advantages of the model:

- *Illustration* of the component effect in a complex network.
- *Facilitated anamnesis collection:* Provides impulses to consider and analyse these components and their mutual influence/control.
- *Assistance in therapy planning*: From the visible networking of the active components of fear, conclusions for therapy planning can be more easily derived.

4.3.2.1 Anxiety Consists of a Network of Active Factors

There are different forms and components of anxiety behaviour. However, these do not each act independently of the others. That is, they act overall as a system or network of fear into the various components and influence each other in the increase of fear with its very diverse manifestations.

Especially in the practice of diagnostics, the seven components of anxiety have proven to be particularly important (Kossak 1993, 2015; Kossak and Zehner 2011). While each of these components has its typical effects, it additionally exerts these effects on the other components through its networking. These effects vary in strength depending on the history, triggering experience, and current situation and are evaluated differently by the individual.

4.3.2.2 The Seven Behavioural Components of Anxiety with their Individual Manifestations and Effects (see Fig. 4.1)

4.3.2.2.1 Emotion

- *Fear as a feeling:* Fears, apprehensions, rejections. Mostly as fear of or at something. Here, the language meaning that has existed for many centuries becomes apparent, as fear comes from the Indo-European *anghu "constricted*", closely related to Latin *angustus/angustina narrowness, constriction, distress.*

4.3.2.2.2 Physiology

- Stress reactions: Release of adrenaline
- *Sympathetic activation*: Increase in heart rate and blood pressure, pallor or blushing

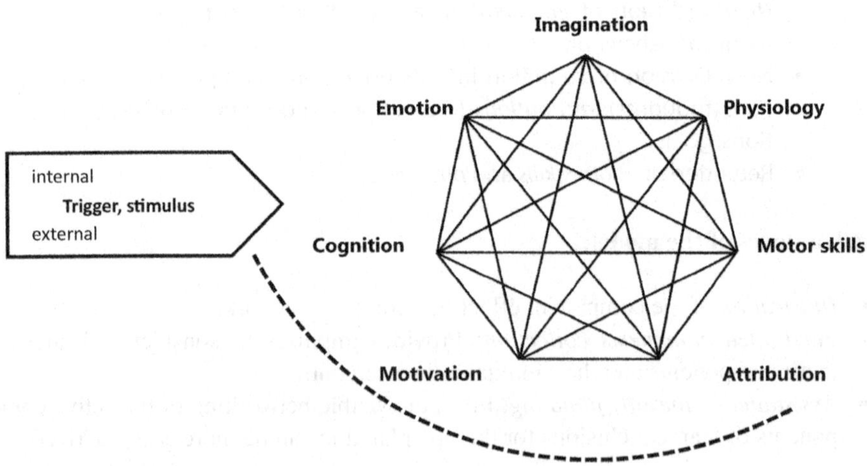

Fig. 4.1 The seven behavioural components of anxiety acting in a network
The original "classical" three *factors cognition, motor skills, and physiology* are supplemented by the factor *emotion* and *imagination*. The factor *cognition* is expanded by *motivation and attribution*—illustrated here as a dotted line.

- Energy supply to the muscles
- Shallow and rapid breathing
- Increased sweat secretion, associated with the release of odours that can be detected by other people and animals, unconsciously triggering alertness in them (Mujica-Parodi et al. 2009).
- *Parasympathetic activation:* Increased stomach and intestinal motility, diarrhoea, nausea, vomiting, urge to urinate

4.3.2.2.3 Motor Skills

- Typical gestures: flight and seeking help, pantomime, facial expressions
- Readiness to flee and flight, overall avoidance behaviour
- Voice trembling, altered voice pitch, rapid, quiet speech
- Hand trembling—possible freezing or loss of tone, weak knees
- Motor tension, restlessness, fidgety movements

Various behaviours can occur in acute fear situations (see below):

- Submission—"*I surrender—I will do anything you want.*"
- Escape—running away, postponing an exam, dropping out of school.
- Playing dead reflex—tension, speech inhibition, mental block "board in front of the head" (rarely occurs in reality).
- Aggression—as a defence mechanism, verbal, physical—e.g. attack on the examiner.

4.3.2.2.4 Cognitions

- Expectations regarding the real or imagined situation: "*The dog is going to approach me*"—"*The dog is looking at me angrily; he wants something from me.*"
- Possible increase in worrisome and negative thoughts, leading to catastrophising: "*If I cannot do this, everyone will laugh at me, it will be in the newspaper, everyone will know that I have NN fear...*"
- Dysfunctional thoughts: "*I will then become impoverished, people will avoid me.*"
- Automatic thoughts about the fear situation: "*I always think about my maths exam.*"
- Impairment of learning and thinking processes by automatically recurring fear thoughts or physiological fear reactions
- Perceptions are distorted and interpreted: "*That is a big dog with long teeth.*"
- Self-verbalisations: "*I should cross to the other side of the street when I see a dog, because I am a loser.*"—"*I want to stop now and observe how long I can endure the fear in this situation.*"
- Behavioural goals (realistic/unrealistic): "*I will confront the boss like Superman.*"

4.3.2.2.5 Attribution—Evaluations

- *Self-evaluation: "I am a failure"—"I rarely succeed at anything"—"I should run away ..."*
- *Evaluation by others:* real or (mostly) only suspected attributions: "*He is a dud*"—"*He is a failure*"—"*He does not succeed at anything.*"—"*I would have wished for a more successful daughter.*"

4.3.2.2.6 Motivation, Expectations, and Goals

- Preferences: "*I want to get out of here; this makes no sense;* I am giving up on school."—"I will never go there again."—"I would rather do something else now."
- Interest/Disinterest: "*I would have liked to become NN.*"—"*That is not for me.*"
- Here, possibly, the questions about the personal resources for coping with fear begin.

4.3.2.2.7 Imaginations

- Imaginations, inner images—(seeing, hearing, smelling, tasting, touching ...) related to objects of fear or fear situations, which can often be very vivid and also unrealistic, such as: "*Then I am hanging with my fear of flying outside at 1000 m altitude on the landing gear and I am helpless.*"

4.4 Practical Tips for Exploration and Diagnosis of Anxiety

Especially with very "clear" anxiety behaviors and their triggers, it can become very tempting to focus only on them. The individual processing possibilities of fear and their effects in the overall network of physiological and psychological can provide valuable diagnostic clues that need to be considered in the exploration.

4.4.1 Subjective Processing Possibilities of Anxiety

In the exploration, one may encounter contradictory statements from the patient. These were not necessarily expressed willingly. Since feelings of fear and their effects are unpleasant, they also touch on self-esteem. Accordingly, the affected person tries to process and describe their experience of fear in different ways.

Cognitive Attitude Tendencies and Strategies of the Individual in Dealing with Fear

- *Coping:* One tries to show an inconspicuous level of anxiety, so that one appears normal and does not deviate from the norm or environmental expectations.

- *Avoidance behavior*: One avoids situations, stimuli, people, events associated with or suspected of fear. These are: silence, running away, not approaching, not thinking about it. In hypnosis, avoid other, harmless, imaginations.
- *Trivializing*: The feelings of fear experienced as embarrassing for the individual are played down in front of them and other people as if they were meaningless.
- *Repression*: One tries to suppress or push away the feelings of fear associated with a task.
- *Denial:* Signs of fear are blocked out of consciousness. As perceived weakness, they can also be hidden, concealed from others.
- *Exaggeration:* The measures perceived or recommended for fear reduction are repeated excessively often and exaggerated. This probably also includes caricaturing one's fear as in a comic, in order to operationalize the fear and supposed fear coping as a possibility of recognition.
- *Generalization*: The experience of anxiety is presented as "normal" and applicable to all, in order to reduce one's experienced or real special position.
- *Heroization*: The emotions of fear are accepted or even sought out in order to experience oneself as a hero or to be perceived as such by the environment.

Without considering this background knowledge, the exploration will contain very altered, thus false information, from which misleading conclusions would be drawn.

4.4.2 Guidelines for Exploration

During a *quiet conversation situation*, the client will feel safe, take more time, and report about themselves in a more detailed manner. As in many areas of experience, confrontation and narration bring about the memory of the event and the associated experiences, triggers, etc. These can then be used in therapy.

- Particularly during the exploration, attention should be paid to the *aspects of VAKOG* and the seven factors presented here.
- The patient will then more easily report their potential coping mechanisms for anxiety problems (see above).

Finding Triggers of Behavioural Chains

Depending on the object of fear (person, situation, etc.) and possibly also on the individual reaction type in these situations, the trigger of a long chain within the effect system would have been very different back then—just as it is in the present. The art of exploration and anamnesis collection is now to find *the initial trigger of this behavioural chain.* If this fortunate case should occur, even the treatment with the effect reduction of this primary component might be sufficient to collapse and render ineffective the chain that has followed it so far and thus the entire effect system of fear. However, this is not always successful.

So we should focus on the effect factors experienced by the patient as the strongest and start therapy here. Experience shows that the other factors in the system are influenced by the reduction of these main effect factors and significantly reduce their subjective effect.

4.4.3 The Anxiety Components as Triggers in the Network—Examples

The seven-component model used here shows the effects of the individual components in their network. To illustrate this, practical examples follow.

The example does not show that these sequences do not occur in a temporally comprehensible order, but possibly within milliseconds.

In the ICD-10, the consequences of fear are very abstractly represented. The concrete effects are manifold and differentiated.

Some Short Examples

The following examples are intended to concretise the diversity of the fear-triggering stimuli and their very different reactions, sequelae, and attempts to cope. This is followed by considerations of a possible prognosis if the disorder continues without therapy. The therapy suggestions that follow are also ideal-typical interventions that are intended to briefly outline the basic treatment options of cognitive-behavioural short-term therapy with hypnosis. This should hopefully make it clear that the method usually works in a short time and permanently, but only if the complex background of the disorder is taken into account—and its complexity within the system of emotion, physiology, imagination, etc. works.

If readers are not familiar with cognitive-behavioural diagnostics and therapy planning, I ask them to refer to Chap. 8.

Case Study 2—Anxiety of Dogs

Clinical Picture

The client sees a dog, notices that he becomes afraid, accompanied by palpitations and accelerated breathing. He wants to escape this aversive situation and crosses to the other side of the street. Simultaneously, he imagines that many people are watching him. He assumes that "the others" are laughing at him—and labels himself a wimp because he is afraid of such a small dog—and feels ashamed. This assumed external evaluation, in turn, generates social anxiety.

Through avoidance behavior (walking away), running away is negatively reinforced, as the client thereby reduces his fear and arousal. However, his negative self-assessment and the anticipated external attribution, followed by shame, remain (see Fig. 4.2).

Stimulus – and its subsequent chain of behavior →

Stimulus – Emotion – Physiology – Motivat. – Motor skills – Imaginat. – Attribution – Emotion

S ------ R -- S ----- R-- S ----------R -- S ---- R -- S ------- R-- S -------- R -- S ----------- R

See dog	Fear	Palpitations Breath	run away	go away	Many see me	"Others laugh". "I am a wimp"	Shame

Fig. 4.2 Fear of dogs involves triggering a chain of behavior
The sight of the dog (S) triggers the other anxiety components of the network. The learning history and subsequent experiences determine how one reacts to an experience (stimulus).

Prognosis
Through the assumed external attribution and shame, a reaction generalization can occur, i.e., the client will either soon take other routes without dogs and people (Is this always possible?) or he will increasingly avoid public routes and potentially suffer secondary disorders: self-doubt, fear of the public, social isolation, depression, etc.

Therapy
Short-term therapy is suitable here, in which the sight of the dog is to be endured and through counterconditioning (see Sect. 8.3.2) the fear is reduced. As a result, his own and external attributions are immediately baseless, as is his shame about it. His behavioral scope is expanded again, thereby increasing his social contact possibilities and his self-confidence. His self-esteem is restored.

Follow-up
Report of freedom from fear even decades later. ◄

Case Study 3—Anxiety of Flying

Clinical Picture
The client becomes afraid and nervous with a fluttering stomach when thinking about an upcoming flight, a situation referred to as . To calm herself, she engages in physical activities such as washing dishes and dusting. She imagines being in a confined airplane with the doors closing. As she desires to fly with her children, she perceives herself as a poor role model for fear management, leading to feelings of guilt (see Fig. 4.3).

Stimulus – and its subsequent chain of behavior ➡

Cognition – Emotion – Physiology – Imagin. – Emot. – Motor skills attribute. – Cognition

S ----------R -- S --------R -- S --------R -- S ---R – S --- R -- S -----R-- S ------------ R

Think about flight	Fear	Being nervous	Flight, Close narrow doors	Fear	Activities	I am: a Anxiety role model, bad Mother	guilty conscience

Fig. 4.3 Individual behavioural components of fear of flying
The thought of the flight triggers other fear components of the network, leading to feelings of guilt towards the children.

Prognosis
This situation may lead her to continue seeking intense physical activities for fear management, potentially developing into compulsive behaviour. Alternatively, she may compensate for her guilt by becoming overprotective of her children, a form of to manage her guilt.

Therapy
Therapy should begin with addressing the initial cognitions, followed by physiological relaxation techniques to reduce overactivity. It is crucial to reduce the cognitions, for instance, (see Sect. 8.3.2) with further relaxation and imagined fear-reducing activities on the plane. As her fear decreases, she will increasingly become a model for fear management for her children. Given her tendency to be overactive, she can utilise this by helping the children pack their suitcases. This activity improves her self-perception as a good and helpful mother, reducing her overall arousal level. Consequently, her negative self-assessment as a "mother" improves, her fear level decreases, and the lose their negative meaning. This reduction in cognitions leads her to think less about the flight or the fear of flying. ◄

In Chap. 11, the topic of fear of flying is presented in detail in Case 11 (see Sect. 12.3.4) and Case 12 (see Sect. 12.3.5).

Case Study 4—Exam Anxiety

State of Affairs
The student suddenly visualizes the scenario "in front of her eyes" where she is in the exam and the professor is asking difficult questions. Consequently, she experiences stomach cramps and thinks: "*I hope I know this.*" Doubts about her self-assessment arise, "*Am I too stupid*?" and she now experiences fear and anxiety about the exam. This motivates her to study more (see Fig. 4.4).

Stimulus – and its consequences ➡

Imaginat. – Physiology – Cognition – Attribution – Emotion – Motivation

S ----------- R --	S ------- R --	S --------- R --	S ------- R --	S --------- R
Examination Heavy Questions	Stomach pressure	I hope I know that.	Am I too stupid?	Fear Fear

	Learn more!!!

Fig. 4.4 The imagination of the exam situation triggers the other anxiety components of the network, leading to the decision to study more.

Prognosis

The result may seem positive at first glance, as she is now studying more. However, learning under the motivation of fear is not always sensible or as successful as desired. Therefore, an analysis of learning and working behaviour should be carried out to determine if learning is effective and efficient. This also includes exploring learning motivation.

Therapy

If she studies well and the fear affects her, the fear-triggering negative imaginations should be reduced in hypnosis by the student recognizing and appreciating the effectiveness of her learning (= cognitive restructuring). If inappropriate because learning is too time-consuming, training in academic and efficient learning behaviour should take place here (see Kossak 2016), after which security occurs and the negative imaginations, followed by fear etc., decrease in favour of self-efficacy. ◄

4.4.4 Effects of Anxiety in Learning and School

4.4.4.1 Generalizations

To illustrate the systemic effect of anxiety, here are a few examples from the learning and school area.

Negative self-concepts impact school performance and exam anxieties (Schilling et al. 2005), thus a low ability self-concept after failures significantly worsens concentration performance (Eckert et al. 2006). People with a high self-concept make an optimistic and positive attribution of their performance and show less avoidance behaviour in learning (Lazarus 2007).

Achievement motivation is closely related to learning and performance emotions, as well as emotions in the intake phase of learning (Laukenmann et al. 2003). Cognitions such as self-concept, self-efficacy beliefs, and willingness to make an effort promote performance (Götz, Zirngibl and Pekrun 2004) or inhibit it.

4.4.4.2 Common Consequences of Anxiety and/or Failure in School, Learning, and Performance Area

- *Stimulus generalization* and *response generalization* leading to helplessness and depression (Seligman 1983).
- *Avoidance behaviour* includes: Delaying the start of work, skipping school, dropping out of a profession or studies, refusing to perform, etc.

For more on the development of fears, see Sect. 6.1.

References

Beck AT (1963) Thinking and depression I. Ideosyncratic content and cognitive distorsions. Arch Gen Psychiatry 9:324–333

Beck AT (1967) Kognitive Therapie der Depression. PVU, Weinheim

Borkovec TD, Wilkinson L, Folensbee R, Lerman C (1983) Stimulus control applications to the treatment of worry. Behav Res Ther 21:247–251

Eckert C, Schilling D, Stiensmeier-Pelster J (2006) Einfluss des Fähigkeitsselbstkonzepts auf die Intelligenz- und Konzentrationsleistung. Zeitschrift für Pädagogische Psychologie 20(1–2):41–48

Ellis A (1994) Reason and emotion in psychotherapy: comprehensive method of treating human disturbances: revised and updated. Citadel Press, New York

Flick SN, Roy-Byrne PP, Cowley DS, Shores MM, Dunner DL (1993) DSM-III-R Personality disorders in a mood and anxiety disorders clinic: prevalence, comorbidity, and clinical correlates. J Affect Disord 27(2):71–79

Götz T, Zirngibl A, Pekrun R (2004) Lern- und Leistungsemotionen von Schülerinnen und Schülern. In: T. Hascher (Hrsg) Schule positiv erleben. Ergebnisse und Erkenntnisse zum Wohlbefinden von Schülerinnen und Schülern, Bern, Haupt, S 49–66

Internationale statistische Klassifikation der Krankheiten und verwandter Gesundheitsprobleme 10. Revision. ICD-10. Dilling H, Mombour W, Schmidt MH (Hrsg) (2019) German Modification, Version 2020. Hogrefe, Göttingen

Jacobi F, Höfler M, Strehle J et al (2014) Psychische Störungen in der Allgemeinbevölkerung Studie zur Gesundheit Erwachsener in Deutschland und ihr Zusatzmodul Psychische Gesundheit (DEGS1-MH). Nervenarzt 85(1):77–87

Kessler RC, Berglund P, Demle O, Jin R, Merikangas KR, Walters EE (2005a) Lifetime prevalence and age-of-onset distributions of DSM-IV disorders in the National Comorbidity Survey Replication. Arch Gen Psychiatry 62(6):593–602

Kessler RC, Demler O, Frank RG et al (2005b) Prevalence and treatment of mental disorders, 1990 to 2003. N Engl J Med 352(24):2515–2523

Kossak H-C, Zehner G (2011) Hypnose beim Kinderzahnarzt. Verhaltensführung und Kommunikation. Springer, Berlin

Kossak H-C (1989) Hypnose. Ein Lehrbuch. Psychologie Verlags Union, München

Kossak H-C (1993) Hypnose. Ein Lehrbuch für Psychotherapeuten und Ärzte, 2. überarb. Aufl., Beltz, PVU, Weinheim

Kossak H-C (2015) Patienteninformationen zur Hypnose. In: Stavemann HH (Hrg) Therapie-Tools. Integrative KBT. 3. Aufl. Beltz. Weinheim, S 648-673

Kossak H-C (2016) Lernen leicht gemacht. Gut vorbereitet und ohne Prüfungsangst zum Erfolg. Carl Auer Systeme, Heidelberg

Lang (1968). Angstminderung und Angstverhalten: Probleme bei der Behandlung eines Konstrukts. In: Shlien JM (Hrsg) Research in psychotherapy, Bd. 3, American Psychological Association, Washington, DC, S 90–102

Laukenmann M, Bleicher M, Fuß S, Gläser-Zikuda M, Mayring P, von Rhöneck C (2003) An investigation of the influence of emotional factors on learning in physics instruction. Int J Sci Educ 25(4):489–507

Lazarus S (2007) Motivation und Leistung: Die Bedeutung von Attribution, Bewertung und Zielorientierung. Dissertation, Ludwig Maximilian-Universität München

Meichenbaum D (1985/2003) Intervention bei Stress. Anwendung und Wirkung des Stressimpfungstrainings. Huber, Bern

Mujica-Parodi LR, Strey HH, Frederick B, Savoy R, Cox D, Botaow J, Tolkunov D, Rubin D, Weber J (2009) Chemosensory cues to conspecific emotional stress activate amygdala in humans. PLoS ONE 4:e6415

Nesse RM (2001) The smoke detector principle. Ann New York Acad Sci 935:75–85

Salkovskis PM (1991) The importance of behaviour in the maintenance of anxiety and panic: A cognitive account. Behav Psychother 19(1):6–19

Schilling SR, Sparfeldt JR, Prusiken C (2005) Aktuelle Aspekte pädagogisch-psychologischer Forschung. In: Schilling SR, Sparfeldt JR, John M (Hrsg) Besser in Mathe—besorgter in Deutsch? Beziehungen zwischen Schulleistungen, schulischen Selbstkonzepten und Prüfungsängsten im Rahmen des I/E-Modells, Beck-shop-de, S 159–178

Seligman MEP (1983) Helplessness. On depression, development, and death. San Francisco: Freeman, 1979 (dt.: Erlernte Hilflosigkeit, 2. Aufl., Urban & Schwarzenberg, München)

Warwitz SA (2016) Formen des Angstverhaltens. In: Ders.: Sinnsuche im Wagnis. Leben in wachsenden Ringen, 2. erw. Aufl., Schneider-Verlag, Hohengehren, S 34–39

Wells A (2011) Kognitive Therapie der Angststörungen. dgvt-Verlag, Tübingen

Neuropsychology of Fear

5

Contents

For the preservation of the species or survival of the individual, the organism must be able to distinguish dangerous stimuli from safe ones. Therefore, learning must occur, after which the individual can distinguish certain stimuli in its environment as dangerous or safe. Accordingly, it must be able to predict the danger that may be associated with certain stimuli. If this learning mechanism, specifically testing stimuli for their outcome, is not present, the organism reacts to many stimuli and situations in general with anxiety or avoidance behaviour, which can lead to pathological anxiety. Extensive neuronal networks and structures are involved in these processing and learning processes, especially the amygdala, the thalamus, the hippocampus, and the prefrontal cortex (see Fig. 5.1).

H.-C. Kossak, *Cognitive-behavioral Psychotherapy for Anxiety*,
https://doi.org/10.1007/978-3-662-69099-4_5

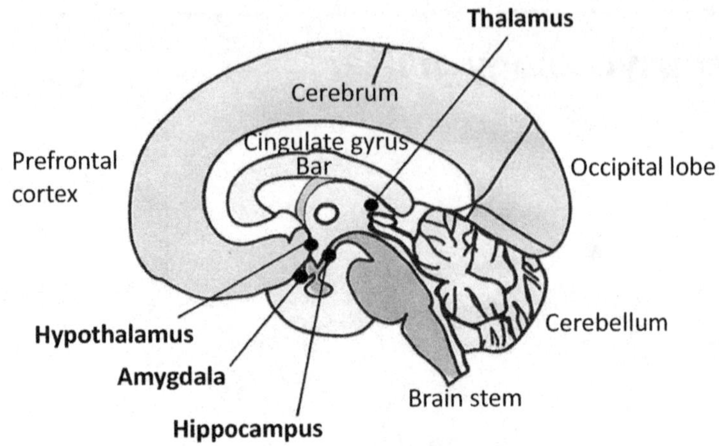

Fig. 5.1 Brain, sagittal sectionThe brain with its areas or functional areas primarily relevant to fear: thalamus, amygdala, hypothalamus, hippocampus, and prefrontal cortex

5.1 The Main Brain Areas Involved in Fear

Essentially, five main areas are of importance in the triggering and processing of fear.

5.1.1 Amygdala (Almond Kernel, Corpus Amygdaloideum)

As a double nucleus, the amygdala is part of the endbrain. Here, sensory information from numerous brain regions converges, such as from the thalamus, hippocampus, and cortex. Signals of sensory perceptions such as seeing, tasting, hearing, feeling also enter here from many cortex areas.

The function of the amygdala is the evaluation of memory performances such as the memory with emotional contents and thus the emergence of feelings of fear, anger, joy.

It evaluates incoming signals and passes them on to the cerebral cortex through its central networking with numerous brain regions. In situations of stress, for example, neurotransmitters such as adrenaline are released, informing the body that a dangerous or important situation is present. The amygdala evaluates this input by comparing it with its memories and then signals whether danger is present; if so, fear arises and the entire organism reacts with increased alertness and possibly with flight reactions. With a "positive evaluation" of the inputs, the sexual drive and reproduction are activated. In American usage, the 4 Fs are managed here (easy to remember): Fear, Fight, Flight, and F… Sexual behavior (Sapolsky 2018).

With frequent fear events, the trigger threshold for these stimuli decreases and causes a stimulus generalization. The amygdala is then overexcited and triggers in similar situations (often unconscious) memories of the primary event and thus reactions such as fear, panic, nausea, without the person being able to assign them to an event.

If the fear is associated with stimuli previously experienced as positive, the memory of the formerly aversive stimulus can be erased, which is referred to as counterconditioning (Kandel et al. 2000; see Sect. 8.3.2).

5.1.2 Thalamus

Consisting of specific nuclei, the thalamus is located in the diencephalon, is partly fused with the hypothalamus and is one of the largest and most differentiated nuclear accumulations of the central nervous system. As a gateway to consciousness, all sensory impressions such as seeing, hearing, etc. enter it (except for the sense of smell) and are distributed and filtered on the way to the cerebral cortex. The thalamus decides which of these come into consciousness and which are forwarded to further switching centers. It also filters what is important for the organism at the moment, i.e., what is a priority, in order to match this with the overall situation such as mating, sleep. The thalamus regulates higher mental activities, such as cognitive and emotional functions. Thalamus and amygdala are virtually parallel in their inputs.

5.1.3 Hypothalamus

The hypothalamus is considered the most important control center for the internal organs and their functions, as well as biological rhythms. It manages and controls fixed behavioural programs for reproduction, brood care, escape and defence reactions. It also serves as the crucial interface between conscious psychological processes (e.g., emotions) and the associated bodily processes (Schandry 2016; see Fig. 5.2).

5.1.4 Hippocampus

While the amygdala compares and evaluates the emotional content of incoming stimuli, the hippocampus is responsible for their storage, i.e., the memory of them. The hippocampus contains several structures located in the telencephalon, where information from the sensory systems converges and is processed, then sent back by the cortex. The function of the hippocampus is to transport memory contents from short-term to long-term memory. It serves as a kind of working memory, where various memory contents are also coordinated.

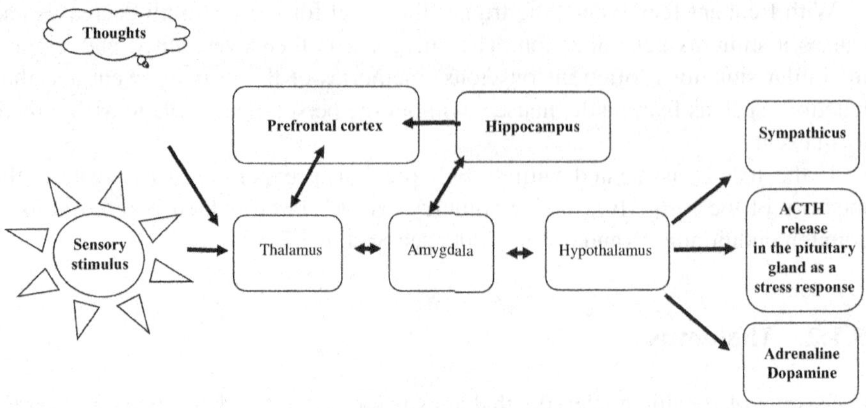

Fig. 5.2 Cooperation of the individual brain areas relevant to fear (simplified block diagram) Incoming external stimuli (sensory stimuli) and internal stimuli (thoughts) are controlled and evaluated by the thalamus and amygdala. They then proceed to the hippocampus and the prefrontal cortex. The hypothalamus is responsible for forwarding them to the body organs.

The hippocampus is one of the few brain areas where new nerve cells can be formed throughout life, which can establish new connections with existing nerve cells (*synaptic plasticity*), i.e., acquisition of new memory contents. The hippocampus is important for the storage and retrieval of learning content. If the learning content located there is unimportant, it is deleted, i.e., forgotten. If the learning content is significant, it is forwarded to the prefrontal cortex.

5.1.5 Prefrontal Cortex

In the anterior brain area, the prefrontal cortex long-term storage takes place. The individual memory contents are meaningfully connected, so that overarching controlling mental principles such as ethics, morality, and personality are located here, as well as the planning and controlling of meaningful actions (see Fig. 5.2).

5.2 Neuronal Effects of Anxiety—Cognitive Blockade

In addition to the many neuronal effects of fear outlined above, its impairing and blocking effect in fear or stress should be mentioned. Under these conditions, the amygdala must quickly and reliably provide escape programs, for example, and use the capacity of the hippocampus working memory for this purpose. All other higher functions are now secondary. Thus, the amygdala blocks the working memory and higher cognitive functions for its use. These are useless, possibly even disruptive, in acute danger (see Fig. 5.3).

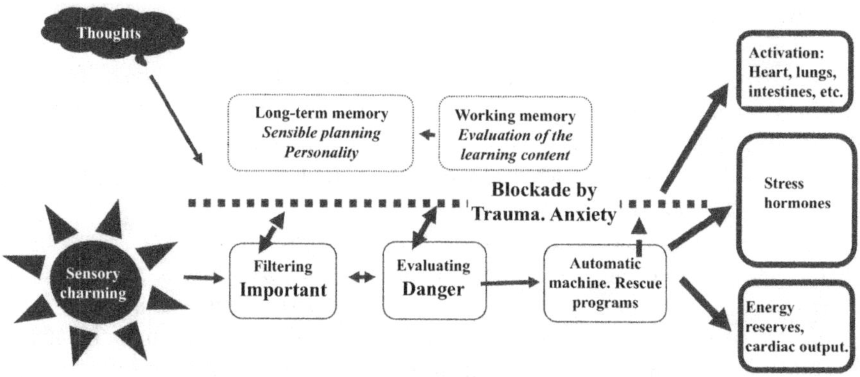

Fig. 5.3 Function of the individual brain areas in fear (simplified block diagram)
If external or internal stimuli are evaluated as dangerous (black), then automatic rescue and escape programs are activated and there is a blockade of higher (cognitive) functions.

5.2.1 Effects of Stress and Fear

Stress and fear desynchronize the activation in various regions of the prefrontal cortex and interrupt the signal connection from the hippocampus to the prefrontal cortex. Due to stress and fear, the hippocampus is "dominated" by the amygdala, whereby fear associations are learned and stored in long-term memory. These in turn increase the excitability of the amygdala via glucocorticoids (see Fig. 5.3). This shows that stress makes it difficult to unlearn fear (Sapolsky 2018).

5.2.2 Archaic Fear Reactions—Comparative Behavioural Research

In instances of strong tension, such as those which arise under high stress and fear (e.g., during exams), the individual is naturally predisposed to these archaic reaction patterns. Many such stress and fear situations are characterized by fear on one side and aggression on the other; it is often a typical conflict situation in which the response is very different and archaic (Eibl-Eibesfeldt 1997). Here, the stimuli coded by the amygdala and thalamus as stress, threat, anxiety are responded to very differently through fixed programs via the hypothalamus:

- *Confusion* – Haphazard, not always controlled and logical behaviour. Mixing up content, sentences, and words. This usually subsides after the first few minutes of experiencing fear, especially when the causes are removed, particularly when calmed down.
- *Submission*—Passive behaviour, avoiding conflicts; e.g., "I'll do whatever you want.—Please spare me."

- *Playing dead*—Motor fright reaction; e.g., "*I am not present and therefore do not provoke an attack.*"
- *Embarrassment*—often manifests itself with archaic behaviours from the grooming and body care area: scratching, especially in the beard or on the head, arranging hair, fiddling with clothing, yawning, stretching.
- *Escape*—Running away, leaving the conflict field; "*I am avoiding the danger.*" Leaving the exam or even not showing up.
- *Aggressions*—Defensive behaviour; "*Attack is the best defence.*" e.g., insulting the opponent (e.g., examiner), threatening him with blows, provoking, etc. *Mini-aggressions* in children are: biting lips, hyperactivity, nail-biting, shouting, destroying objects. These behaviours are relatively common in anxious children, e.g., during a dentist visit (Kossak and Zehner 2011).

The acquired social control of the prefrontal cortex usually dictates to react appropriately in the situation. However, this may not always be successful depending on the disposition (e.g., in the case of "father issues") and the accumulation of some unfavourable variables. The cognitive attitude tendencies and strategies in dealing with fear are influenced by these archaic fear reactions and indirectly manifest themselves in the anamnesis (see Sect. 4.4.1.1)

Example: "Father Issues"

A client with "father issues" reacts in the exam due to his socialization with defiant refusal to the professor's questions.

Another client with a different genesis of his "father issues" reacts submissively to the examiner—and yet another with feelings of guilt and embarrassment, etc. ◄

5.2.3 Effects of Cognitive Blockage on Learning and Retention

The effects of this alarm circuit, in connection with anxiety, have been studied extensively (Schandry 2016; Kolb and Whishaw 2019). The following are some of the findings related to cognitive blockage:

- Learning material stored in the hippocampus is automatically removed in instances of anxiety or stress to free up capacity in the working memory.
- Under the influence of learning is often inadequate and yields poor results.
- Cognitive explanations provided during a state of anxiety, such as "This is harmless" or "Handle this math formula differently …" etc., are rarely retained. For instance, a patient experiencing fear and pain in the dentist's chair will likely not remember the dentist's well-intentioned advice (Kossak and Zehner 2011).

- Severe fear, such as that experienced in Post-Traumatic Stress Disorders (PTSD), can affect memory, learning, and concentration.
- It is worth noting that similar cognitive blockages can also occur during advertising and mating behaviour, as these are regulated by similar circuits as fear.

Preliminary Consequences for Anxiety Treatment
From these various biopsychological functions, it can be inferred that a common therapeutic method is to initially focus on calming and relaxation. This approach aims to influence the amygdala in such a way that it becomes "relaxed" and no longer sends out warning signals or triggers escape behaviour. Suitable relaxation methods include autogenic training, progressive muscle relaxation, or hypnosis relaxation.

Subsequently, depending on the specific needs, various intervention methods (with or without hypnosis) such as those for self-control can be implemented.

References

Eibl-Eibesfeldt I (1997) Die Biologie des menschlichen Verhaltens. 3. überarb. Aufl., Seehammer, Wayarn

Kandel ER, Schwartz JH, Jessell TM (2000) Principles of neural science, 4. Aufl. New York, McGraw Hill Medical

Kolb B, Whishaw IO (2019) Fundamentals of human neuropsychology, 7. Aufl. Worth, New York

Kossak H-C, Zehner G (2011) Hypnose beim Kinderzahnarzt. Verhaltensführung und Kommunikation. Springer, Berlin

Sapolsky R (2018) Gewalt und Mitgefühl. Die Biologie des menschlichen Verhaltens (2. Aufl). Hanser, München

Schandry R (2016) Biologische Psychologie, 4. Aufl. Beltz, Weinheim

Learning Theory Paradigms

6

Contents

The short therapy presented here is a combination of hypnosis and cognitive behavioural therapy. As a short therapy, it incorporates numerous elements of these two methods in a condensed form. It should not be thought that the short form is merely symptom manipulation. Therefore, a brief introduction to the relevant learning theories will follow, including a short historical overview of this method combination.

Learning theories posit that behaviour, both normal and abnormal, is learned and can therefore be unlearned using appropriate methods.

H.-C. Kossak, *Cognitive-behavioral Psychotherapy for Anxiety*,
https://doi.org/10.1007/978-3-662-69099-4_6

The methods presented here are merely the fundamental building blocks of diagnostics and therapy. However, behavioural theories and cognitive behavioural therapy consist of many more of these elements. For our purposes, the presentation of the basic theories and methods should suffice, as they are also the main elements of short therapy.

Thus, at least basic experiences in hypnosis and cognitive behavioural therapy are assumed.

As already mentioned in the introduction in Sect. 4.3, we aim to present the theoretical aspects essential in cognitive behavioural therapy for the genesis and maintenance of fears, focusing more on their practical relevance.

6.1 Behavioural theoretical genesis of disorders

With the learning theories, we encounter initial animal experiments, the results of which were then applied to human behaviour. The learning laws derived from this were initially dismissed as rat psychology. Over time, however, it was recognized that these learning laws apply to all living beings. All (higher) living beings have an innate learning disposition (Eibl-Eibesfeldt and Wickler 1962). The conditioned reflex can be observed in the yellow-banded beetle as well as in fish, rats, and monkeys. Learning from success is as effective in toads as it is in fish, turtles, and monkeys. Learning by observation can be demonstrated in squirrels, ravens, dolphins, elephants, and monkeys (Eibl-Eibesfeldt 1967). Only the cognitive-behavioural methods are reserved for hominids, to which we belong.

The presentation of learning theories sometimes gives the impression that they are soulless technical manipulations of people. Their *explanations* are indeed very abstract, referring to concepts, components, dependent and independent variables, etc. Their *implementation*, on the other hand, uses these theoretical structures, but always presupposes empathy, understanding, respect, and often insight of the counterpart (therapist, client, patient, child, etc.).

For our presentation purposes, the sometimes very complex learning theories can only be presented in their essential basic features. Additional theoretical discussions should also be omitted here for simplification.

> **Important**
> The summaries of the learning theories serve as a kind of repetition for those who have had to deal less with them so far. Everyday examples are also inserted for them. Those well-versed in learning theories will probably skip these sections.

6.1.1 The Conditioned Reflex

A widely known example is the "Pavlovian Dog". The Physiologist I.P. Pavlov discovered in 1923 through his experiments with dogs that they could be trained to salivate at the sound of a bell. This means that the otherwise involuntary production of saliva at the sight or smell of food could now be voluntarily triggered by the signal tone. The revolutionary aspect was that it was discovered how a previously insignificant stimulus for the animal (bell sound) could trigger a reflex-like physiological reaction (salivation). This learned process was referred to as a *conditional reflex*. It is not just an artificial reaction created in the lab. In everyday life, the conditional reflex is relatively common.

Example: Classical Conditioning

A person experiences a fright in the dark. This could be due to a tire bursting during an evening walk, witnessing an accident, or a sudden bang in the basement (short circuit, cat knocking a bottle off the shelf, etc.). The simultaneous experience of darkness and fright results in conditioning that now merely perceiving darkness (or thinking about dark rooms, etc.) triggers the fright reaction. From then on, a long-lasting fear of the dark can begin (see Fig. 6.1).

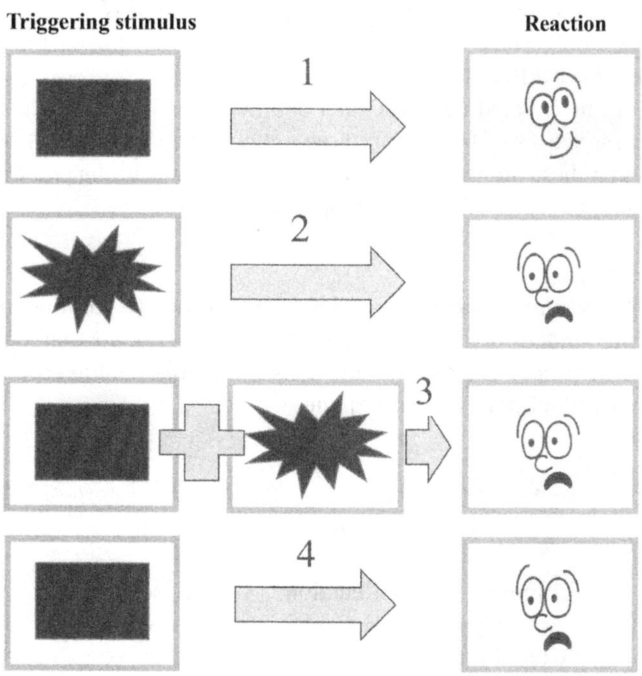

Fig. 6.1 Classical Conditioning—Example. 1. In the previously neutral stimulus situation of darkness, one reacts neutrally-calm. 2. In response to an unexpected loud noise (bang, horn, tire burst, glass break, flash), one naturally reacts reflexively with fright (sweating, etc. = alarm by amygdala). 3. If the loud fright stimulus occurs *during* the darkness, this results in conditioning. 4. The stimulus "darkness" alone (seeing, thinking about it) will soon reflexively trigger the fright reaction: The fear of the dark has been conditioned

If this fear of the dark persists for a long time and remains uncomfortably intense, it can even restrict the affected person's freedom and can be described as a phobia. This is how many fears are created.

A harmless positive everyday example would be that our mouths water when reading the menu—or that we get an appetite just by looking at the restaurant logo (the burger chain, the cookie package, etc.). This is exploited by advertising and special advertising designs. ◄

Many phobias and psychosomatic diseases are usually caused by random classical conditioning. They are often then maintained by attention = "illness gain" operantly (see below).

6.1.2 Operant Learning

In the historical view of learning theories, we encounter Skinner's discovery of operant learning (Skinner 1938). From his animal experiments, it emerged as a law of learning that under a certain stimulus constellation (S), a behaviour (R) is shown more frequently if it receives an immediate reward (C+ = Reinforcement) for it (see Fig. 6.2). Here too, only the basic factors are shown, fully aware that many of them have differentiations.

For a better understanding of the later abbreviations in the sketches of the triggers and consequences of behaviour, these are compiled in Table 6.1. Here it must be clarified that these are the basic elements of operant learning, which were modified depending on further theory development.

> **Important**
> The *immediate* reward of the relevant behaviour (= contingency) is absolutely necessary (= contingent reinforcement), so that only *the desired behaviour* is precisely and differentiatedly reinforced and not another, just randomly occurring one.

S ----------	R ---------	C+
Stimulus	Reaction	Consequence
Antecedence	Behavior	Consequence
Cue Stimulus		

Fig. 6.2 Operant Reinforcement.
A certain stimulus (S) triggers a behaviour (R). If it is followed by a positive consequence (C +), it is thereby more frequent = positively reinforced. The representation of this basic process is greatly simplified

Table 6.1 Basic terms of operant learning—S—R—C

Symb.	Explanation	Naming	Effects on behavior
C +	The behavior is followed by a **positive** consequence.	**Positive reinforcement,** reward (e.g. praise, attention, treats)	**Increase** the frequency
C -	The *consequences* of a behavior are **negative**, *unpleasant, aversive.*	**Direct punishment** (e.g. blows, pain).	**Decrease** of frequency
~~C~~ +	As a consequence of the behavior, a positive consequence is removed (reinforcement withdrawal).	**Indirect punishment** (e.g. love deprivation)	**Decrease** of frequency
~~C~~ -	The behavior *ends* an aversive situation.	**Negative reinforcement** (see avoidance behavior)	**Increase** the frequency

Note: The term negative reinforcement is often misunderstood as punishment. "*Negative*" here refers to the removal/termination of an aversive/negative consequence. (*Negative* is therefore not morally judgmental).

Types of reinforcers (partly culturally, socially, economically determined)
social: attention, smiles, praise, promotion, cooperation
verbal: praise, recognition, grades
cognitive: self-praise, self-reinforcement, positive thoughts
material: money, toys, objects, gold, jewelry
nutritive: nutrition, treats, favorite food, drinks
sexual: drive satisfaction (in various forms)

Types of reinforcement
continuous: always
intermittent: occasionally, randomly
planned: randomly according to certain *rules*

Sources of reinforcement
extrinsic = *externally* mediated by a person (partner, therapist)
intrinsic = *self* through self-reward/self-reinforcement/self-praise/satisfaction etc.

Example: Reinforcement of undesired behaviour

Sometimes inappropriate or pathological behaviours can also be caused by operant reinforcement. In the following example, a fear of dogs arises, not through instrumental learning (see above), but through operantly reinforced attention (see Fig. 6.3). ◄

Everyday examples

Many of our everyday behaviours are learned operantly: writing, reading, speaking, using tools, riding a bicycle, etc., as well as fears.

Reinforcements can be: attention, treats, good body feelings (like stroking), school grades, money, but also praise, recognition.

	S	R	C+
Child:	The sight of a dog	Crying	Attention from the mother

Fig. 6.3 Fear caused by operant reinforcement. The child sees a dog and then cries (because: it is frightened, the dog is unknown, etc., randomly). The mother immediately comforts the child. Since the mother gives the child attention in this situation, she can thereby reinforce her child's crying, i.e., make it more frequent when it will see a dog in the future. This made the development of an operantly reinforced fear possible

These reinforcements must be *contingent*, i.e., immediate, so that now the behaviour just shown is built up and not another unwanted one that randomly occurs in between (see above). In this way, the therapist reinforces the patient's cooperation. Even the smallest reactions that go in the desired direction must be reinforced in this way until finally a complex—and relevant for hypnosis—behaviour is present.

In the further development of behaviour therapy, the effectiveness of social and cognitive variables or reinforcers in the emergence and maintenance of behaviours was also recognized.

> **Important**
> In everyday reality, mixed forms of, for example, instrumental and operant learning processes can sometimes be found.
> The determining factors such as attribution, emotion, motivation, and imagination continue to be decisive.

6.1.3 Learning by Observation—Model Learning—Imitation Learning

Bandura (1969) found in his experimental study on children that many behaviours are learned through observing other people, referred to as models. These models can act as causes of anxiety, but they can also be used in the treatment of fears.

Case Study 5—Vertigo

Clinical Picture

Mrs. K., 37 years old, seeks therapy for her 14-year-old daughter, Mechthild, an 8th-grade high school student, who suffers from a severe fear of heights and is generally quite insecure. She does not have other problems, for example, in social areas at school.

History

In histories, it is always important to ask if a family member or person in the immediate social environment has similar problems to those mentioned, in order to consider possible model learning.

The mother reports that as a child during the war, she had to flee across a narrow bridge over an abyss while being shot at by fighter planes. She describes it as "like in a creepy spy movie". The daughter appears open-minded, but slightly insecure, especially when she has to perform an exercise in front of all her classmates in sports. In addition, she has a fear of heights.

Diagnosis

Mother and daughter act as model persons for fear behaviour on each other and favour unsuccessful fear coping.

Prognosis

This mutual model effect creates a permanent maintenance of anxiety. Without appropriate treatments, the fear of heights, followed by the daughter's insecurity, will continue.

Therapy Planning and Implementation

Subsequently, the decision is made to include the mother in the treatment; since she acted as a model for fear behaviour, she should now serve as a model for fear reduction by sharing her successes with her daughter. Parallel to this, the daughter is advised on how to better cope with her insecurities. With the mother, a desensitization in hypnosis takes place, in which fear imaginations of increasing strength alternate with relaxation scenes.

After about three sessions, the mother surprisingly comes to the appointment together with her daughter. Beaming with joy, she tells that they went for coffee last weekend: in the rotating café of the Dortmund television tower at about 200 m height! They enjoyed the beautiful view with coffee and cake (= counter-conditioning). The therapy plan was thus realized faster than ever thought—and mother and daughter remained free of fear.

Follow-up

Even after many years, these positive changes in mother and daughter have remained stable. ◄

Everyday Examples

Many of our desired or undesired behaviours are learned operantly or through model effect like, for example, table manners, dealing with morality, truth, justice, motivation—as well as anxieties. Often children with anxiety problems are presented, which were caused by their mothers as fear role models. The influencers appearing in the media are particularly strong models for imitation of fashion, consumption and attitudes.

6.1.3.1 Factors and Characteristics of Frequently Copied Models

The detailed research according to Bandura shows that people (= models) are most often imitated when they exhibit certain characteristics:

- Same age, gender, assumed similarity (peer group)
- Power, dominance, high status (family members)
- Competence
- Enthusiasm, friendliness (e.g. teachers)
- Having success, receiving reward (attention, recognition, status gain. Praise, sweets etc.)

As a result, undesirable behaviours such as gang membership, assaults etc. can also be copied from corresponding models, as they gain recognition and status through their actions, which may be dubious or criminal, but leads to fame in their subculture.

6.1.3.2 Covert Behaviour in Psychotherapy—Hypnosis

All these behaviour therapy methods, including the cognitive-behavioural ones, can be carried out in hypnosis if they are left in their basic functions and adapted to the possibilities of hypnosis, i.e. the area of imaginations. Since this primarily does not involve visible behaviour (overt behaviour), this is also referred to as covert (covert behaviour). In their effects and in therapy practice, they hardly differ according to experience. Hypnosis thus works exclusively with covert, i.e. imagined behaviour.

6.1.4 Learning through Cognitive Changes

Initially, cognitive therapy was introduced with its theories and methods as an independent theory and form of therapy. However, due to practical application, combinations of both forms quickly emerged, complementing each other optimally and yielding very effective therapy results. This functional eclecticism pragmatically led to the creation of the *Cognitive Behavioral Therapy* (CBT)—also known as *Cognitive Behavior Therapy* (CBT).

Numerous new methods were developed in this area. In the context of this book, only the essential ones can be mentioned as pioneers or foundational theories of CBT. These are also the ones that can be particularly easily combined with hypnosis.

Cognitive therapy is particularly used for anxiety disorders, among other things, through Socratic dialogues, Reframing, confrontation with anxiety, and reduction of safety behavior, stress inoculation trainings (Meichenbaum 1986).

6.1.4.1 The Cognitive Model of Ellis

Simplified, the model of Ellis (1970) posits that interpretations and assumptions about a perception determine behavior and feelings (see Fig. 6.4).

A →	B →	C
Activating internal and external events	Assessments Interpretations Assumptions	Consequence Emotion, behavior

Fig. 6.4 The ABC Model of Ellis (Dryden and Ellis 1988). Upon the perception (A) of certain events, these events are individually judged and interpreted. Assumptions about the events (B) arise—and sometimes the entire associated environment. These assumptions influence emotions or motor behavior, further actions and perceptions (C)

During this processing, there can be misconceptions and basic beliefs, the *irrational assumptions,* that govern life.

The irrational assumptions include (Ellis 1970):

- All-or-nothing thinking
- Focusing on negative aspects
- Ignoring positive aspects
- Personalizing
- Perfectionism

6.1.4.2 Cognitive Therapy—Beck's Model (1967)

Beck's model (1967) posits that cognitive aspects are the essential components in the development of depression and other mental/cognitive disorders. These components include *attributions,* or assumptions about causalities, *dysfunctional schemas,* or automatic perspectives, and *cognitive errors,* or specific thought patterns.

Examples: Cognitive Errors (DeRubeis and Beck 1988)

- *Arbitrary conclusions:* symptom-related conclusions drawn without sufficient justification
- *Selective abstraction*: considering only details, without taking into account the relevant context
- *Overgeneralization*: Establishing "universally valid" rules without background information or based on a single (irrelevant) event
- *Personalization*: Relating everything to oneself, without an objective basis
- *Dichotomous thinking*: black-white, all or nothing thinking—without gradations; the patient perceives himself at the negative end of the scale

Everyday examples

Statements and *self-attributions* (self-evaluations) include: "*I am a jinx; I am always disadvantaged; everyone always looks at me with pity; no one notices me.*"

Assumed *external attributions* include: "*They don't like me anyway; they would love to laugh at me; they think I'm a coward.*"

6.1.4.3 Self-instruction training—according to Meichenbaum (1969)

Meichenbaum considers cognitive aspects, including thought processes and *linguistic* processes that control behaviour, as they are accompanying phenomena of human action. Based on developmental psychological observations, he developed the *self-instruction training* method (1986). In children, it is often used for self-control. In adults, it is a component of complex therapy strategies, such as for self-encouragement, motivation, and emotion regulation. Fliegel (1978) uses self-instruction innovatively in the treatment of fears.

6.1.4.4 Self-regulation—Kanfer (1977)

In the further development of what is now referred to as cognitive-behavioral theories and treatment methods, self-regulation and its various aspects are of great importance. This includes the mental management of one's own moods, feelings, and the intentions and abilities to actualize through targeted and reality-related actions (Kanfer et al. 2000).

As seen in model learning, it becomes clear that cognitive processes are central in controlling human behavior. "The role of conscious actions, the conscious experience of conflicts and abilities, to make one's own decisions even against an obvious external control, are decisive principles of self-control." (Reinecker 1999, p. 301). A hierarchy of preferences, goals, and motivational aspirations determines our decisions and actions. If these regulatory processes are impaired by themselves or other symptoms, there are miscontrols that manifest themselves in disorders such as depression, hypochondria, and social anxieties.

6.1.4.4.1 Self-regulation

Self-regulation typically begins when obstacles occur on the way to the desired goal, or when habitual behaviors are disturbed or interrupted. This area also includes: emotion control, impulse control, and frustration tolerance.

6.1.4.4.2 Self-control

Self-control is a specific instance of self-regulation, in which a chain of behavior is interrupted because there is a conflict between two behaviors. The conflicts are either the resistance to a temptation situation or heroic behavior: i.e., carrying out a behavior even though it causes short-term aversive consequences.

6.1.4.4.3 Self-management

Self-management is the ability to change one's own behavior using specific strategies.

6.1.4.5 Further Forms of Cognitive Therapy

Cognitive therapy is particularly used for anxiety disorders, among other things, through Socratic conversations, reframing, anxiety confrontation, and reduction of safety behavior stress inoculation trainings (Meichenbaum 1986).

6.2 Maintenance of Anxiety

Once experienced, fear situations can persist over long periods and, with a certain strength and frequency, can severely restrict a person's behavioral options. In such cases, these are usually so-called phobias: fear of dogs, cats, spiders, dentists, injections, open spaces, tight spaces, crowds, tall buildings, germs, flights, etc.

Fortunately, behavior therapy has developed different explanatory models and treatment methods for this. The most common conditions that can continue to maintain a behavior (here fear) are presented below.

6.2.1 Avoidance Behaviour and Negative Reinforcement

Fears, particularly, can persist for a very long time, over many years, due to . This can be caused, on one hand, by a very strong traumatic experience; on the other hand, often by avoidance behavior. This implies that one does not want to encounter the unpleasant (= aversive) anxiety again, to avoid experiencing fear again. Thus, one avoids such fear-associated situations, i.e., the fear-inducing stimuli. As a result, one naturally feels relief and is glad to have escaped the aversive situation (C-), but the fear is not reduced by this, but rather becomes more frequent (see Fig. 6.5).

> **Avoidance—Often Negative Reinforcement**
> Possible fear situations or aversive stimuli are often avoided.
> The tension level decreases and relaxation sets in by fleeing from it (or avoiding it). This is, of course, very pleasant.

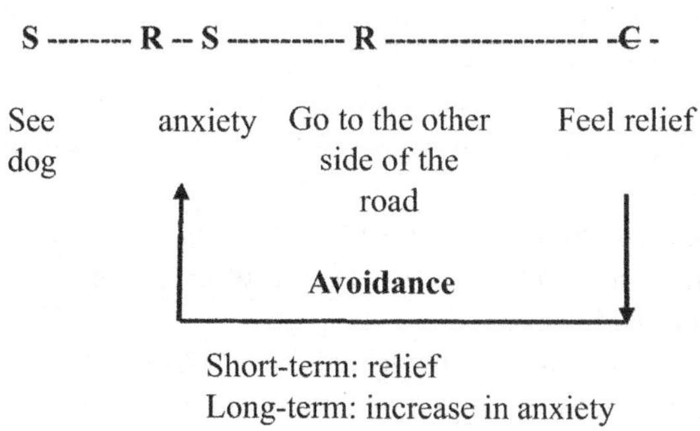

Fig. 6.5 The effect of avoidance behaviour—negative reinforcement—example of fear of dogs. By avoiding the sight of the dog and the resulting fear, the person, for example, crosses to the other side of the street. This reduces their aversive feeling (fear), which provides short-term relief. Therefore, their crossing to the other side of the street will become more frequent: They experience negative reinforcement through the cessation of fear. But in the long term, the fear remains or even increases, as the fear situation continues to be avoided and counter-experiences like "dog is harmless" cannot be made.

Therefore, the avoidance or escape behaviour becomes more frequent, as it is negatively reinforced by the absence of negative consequences.

In addition, a positive counter-experience is not possible due to avoidance learning, namely the triggering stimulus (S = seeing dog) and the fear situation (R) can never be experienced as harmless or neutral. Therefore, many behaviour therapy methods for treating fear aim to reduce and endure the fear. This changes long-established actions and feelings and the previous triggers are experienced as neutral. It is not always easy for patients to interrupt these ingrained fear-laden behaviour patterns, even if they suffer from them.

6.2.2 Operant Reinforcement as a Learning Process Within a System

The example in Fig. 6.5 expands on the operant reinforced dog fear depicted in Fig. 6.3. It demonstrates that operant reinforcement is not merely a one-dimensional reinforcement. Instead, it often involves complex reinforcement systems within a social system.

Evaluation and Additions to the Case Study (Refer to Figs. 6.5 and 6.6)
The following aspects become clear:

- Operant conditioning is never one-sided, as reinforcements are typically provided by social partners such as parents, siblings, peer groups, etc.
- The individuals providing reinforcement have motives for behaving in such a reinforcing manner.
- Emotions, attributions, and motivations as effective factors (stimuli and/or reactions) are significant (see Sect. 5.3.2).
- Since this often involves action within a social system of family, partnership, or friendship, their motives, behaviour, and reinforcements must also be considered.
- For one child, the comforting of a sibling can trigger feelings of neglect, i.e., a perceived deficit of attention (C/+). The child may then develop symptoms to gain attention as well (C+).
- Similarly, a husband may feel neglected (C/+or C-) and become jealous of his child. This could result in aggression towards the child, which could then be superficially dismissed as a father-son problem without investigating the underlying causes.

It becomes clear that in this example the chain of reinforcements must be broken as early as possible:

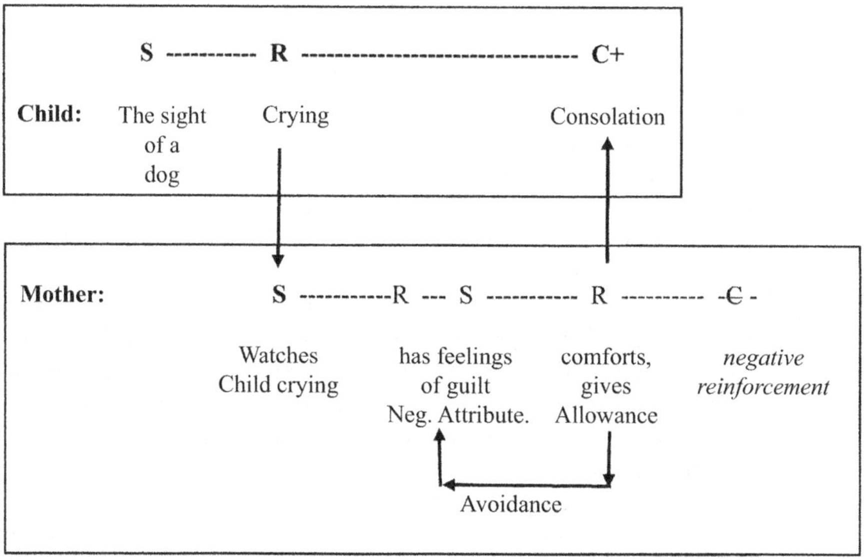

Fig. 6.6 Operant reinforcement of fear in a system—example family. The sequences of individual triggers, behaviours, and reinforcements in the diagram are explained below in their chronological order. 1. The child cries at the sight of a dog. 2. The crying is the stimulus for the mother to feel guilty and to perceive herself as a bad mother. 3. The feelings of guilt trigger the mother to immediately comfort the child. Since the mother gives the child attention in this situation, she can thereby operantly reinforce the child's crying, i.e., make it more frequent when the child sees a dog in the future. 4. The mother avoids the three aversive states of seeing the child cry, having feelings of guilt, and evaluating herself as a bad mother. This is the *negative reinforcement* of her behaviour to continue comforting the child. 5. Thus, the child continues to be reinforced in being afraid of a dog. If a *generalization* occurs, the child will always be tearful or afraid in supposed fear or tension situations or at the sight of animals, fur, etc.

- The mother should be supported by her husband in not feeling guilty when her child cries, but in recognizing the perspective of helping the child by ignoring it (elimination of reinforcement = C/+) and thus reducing the crying = extinction.
- As a result, an emotional deficit arises for the child, and it could now produce other symptoms or behaviours to continue receiving the usual attention.
- Therefore, the child should then receive increased attention and affection for alternative appropriate behaviour = reinforcement.
- If the father supports his wife in this, reinforces her for her changed behaviour, and gives her more partnership attention, this will be easier.
- At the same time, he receives more attention from his wife and the relationship with his son improves, as he no longer has to be jealous of him.

6.2.3 Reinforcement and Learning Processes in a Social System

- Operant reinforcements take place in a social environment where people either provide or withhold reinforcements.
- Individual behaviour is triggered not only by external stimuli (such as seeing, hearing), but also by internal stimuli (like attribution, emotion, motivation).
- Consequently, many communications or behaviours within a social system are regulated, determined, and reinforced.
- Inappropriate reinforcements often lead to avoidance behaviour, which builds and maintains undesirable behaviours (typically behavioural disorders).
- Changes in the treatment of these disorders must occur within the system that triggers and maintains them. This involves engaging the people within this system (parents, siblings, friends, partners, etc.) and altering their behaviour by changing their systems of reinforcement, reward, avoidance, or punishment.
- Overall, this can lead to changes in the entire family and relationship network. The resulting positive and negative consequences and effects should be considered in the treatment process.

Perform Differentiated Diagnostics
In the case of fears, direct behavioural therapeutic treatment of the child can be as effective as special training for their parents (Lebowitz et al. 2020). However, these results should not be generalized, as the causal and maintaining conditions of fears vary greatly. Accordingly, these behavioural contingencies should be clarified through differentiated diagnostics, possibly also through behavioural observations and video recordings. See also case examples 5 (Sect. 6.1.3 fear of heights) and 10 (see Sect. 12.3.3 fear as a victim of a dog attack).

6.2.4 Generalization

Stimulus generalization. Prolonged or intense anxiety confrontation can lead to fear being triggered by an increasing number of stimuli that are similar to the original trigger. For example, not only the dog Pluto triggers the fear, but all dogs, all animals, and even all furry objects—furs, pelts, etc.

Response generalization. The reaction or avoidance reaction increases in strength or frequency. Fear then escalates to panic, leading to anxiety attacks, helplessness, depression (Seligman 1983). Or the avoidance is not only quiet waiting or leaving, but also screaming, crying, running away, etc.

6.2.5 Dyscognitions and Self-Regulation Disorders

With the increasing duration of fear, the associated cognitions can become increasingly negative and increasingly deviate from reality. Such *dyscognitions* can be, for example: "*That is a **dangerous** dog. He looks so bloodthirsty. I wonder if his master has him under control? He can quickly break loose and attack me*!"

Also, *mis-regulations* can occur, which further solidify the disorder, such as in self-assessment or in attempts at compensation.

References

Bandura A (1969) Principles of behavior modification. Holt, Rinehart & Winston, London

Beck AT (1967) Kognitive Therapie der Depression. PVU, Weinheim

DeRubeis RJ, Beck AT (1988) Cognitive therapy. In: KS Dobson (Hrsg) Handbook of cognitive-behavioral therapies, Guilford Press, New York

Eibl-Eibesfeldt I, Wickler WC (1962) Ontogenese und Organisation von Verhaltensweisen. Fortschritte der Zoologie 15:345–377

Eibl-Eibesfeldt I (1967) Grundriss der vergleichenden Verhaltensforschung. Piper, München

Ellis (1970) The essence of rationale psychotherapy: a comprehensive approach to treatment. Institute of Rational Living, New York

Fliegel S (1978) Zur Wirksamkeit von Selbstverbalisationen bei der Verhaltenstherapie phobischer Ängste. Inaugural-Dissertation, Ruhr-Universität Bochum

Kanfer FH (1977) The many faces of self-control, or behavior modification changes ist focus. In RB Stuart (Hrsg.) Behavioral self-management. Brunner/-Mazel, New York, 1–48

Kanfer FH, Reinecker R, Schmelzer D (2000) Selbstmanagement-Therapie, 3. Aufl. Springer, Berlin

Lebowitz ER, Marin C, Martino A, Shimshoni Y, Silverman WK (2020) Parent-based treatment as effiacious as cognitive-behavioral therapy for childhood anxienty: A randomized noninferiority study of supportive parenting for anxious childhood emotions. J Am Acad Child Adolesc Psychiatry 59(3):362–372

Meichenbaum D (1969) The effects of instructions and reinforcement on thinking and language behavior of schizophrenics. Behav Res Ther 7:101–114

Meichenbaum D (1986) Cognitive-behavior modification. In FH Kanfer, AP Goldstein (Hrsg) Helping people change, 3. Aufl., Pergamon Press, New York

Pawlow IP (1923) The identity of inhibition with sleep and hypnosis. Sci Monog 17:603–608

Reinecker H (1999) Grundlagen verhaltenstherapeutischer Methoden. In Reinecker H, Borg-Laufs M, Ehlert U, Schulte D, Sorgatz H, Vogel H (Hrsg) Lehrbuch der Verhaltenstherapie, dgvt-Verlag, Tübingen, S 87–146

Seligman MEP (1983) Helplessness. On depression, development, and death. Freeman, San Francisco: 1975 dt.: Erlernte Hilflosigkeit. 2. Aufl. Urban & Schwarzenberg, München

Skinner BF (1938) The behavior of organisms: an experimental analysis. Appleton-Century Company, New York

Learning Theory Paradigms and Neuropsychology

7

Contents

7.1 Instrumental (Classical) Conditioning

The essential learning process for individual survival is classical instrumental conditioning (Pawlow 1938). This basic form of learning allows living beings to store and encode certain connections between a stimulus and its consequences. This encoding enables them to exhibit appropriate adaptive behaviour in the presence of the stimulus.

In the case of synaptic transmission of conditioned stimuli (CS) to the amygdala, a process known as classical *anxiety conditioning* takes place. During this process, the once neutral avoidance behaviour becomes conditioned behaviour (CR) through a specific synaptic transmission to the amygdala. This results in a certain "input specificity" in stimulus processing, which can serve the selectivity of conditioned fear reactions.

In the case of fear extinction, *extinction learning* can cause the depolarization of synapses altered by conditioning. However, the synapses altered by conditioning continue to maintain their connections (Kim and Cho 2017). This explains the potential risk of relapse if the treated critical behaviour has not been sufficiently stabilized.

H.-C. Kossak, *Cognitive-behavioral Psychotherapy for Anxiety*,
https://doi.org/10.1007/978-3-662-69099-4_7

7.2 Operant Learning—Learning by Success

A network of neuronal connections, primarily located in the prefrontal cortex, responds particularly to dopamine, a neurotransmitter associated with positive feelings and reward.

There is a reward-seeking system, with certain behaviours causing a *dopamine release*. Since there is also a close link with the amygdala and the hippocampus, the results of relevant events are stored in memory. This can explain why a behaviour becomes more frequent through reward and is activated when needed (deficits), i.e., to actively receive rewards again with this typical learned behaviour.

> **Important**
> Stimuli that predict a reward, for example, the anticipation of a reward, already cause the release of dopamine, even if the corresponding event does not occur (Panksepp 2004; Schultz 2006, 2007).

Since this learning is not unconsciously triggered by reflexes (i.e., uncontrollable, immediate), but is used specifically to achieve a positive state, it is also referred to as operant. This includes the fact that pathological behaviours can also arise and be maintained through operant learning processes.

Example: Development of Problem Behaviour through Reinforcement

Secondary defiant behaviour, for example, through attention, secondary gain from illness, for example, through headache, illness, disability receive attention, get advantages, be spared. ◄

7.3 Learning from a Model—Imitation Learning—Observational Learning

The basis for imitation learning is the mirror neurons, a group of nerve cells in the premotor cortex (Rizzolatti and Sinigaglia 2008). In connection with other regions, including the amygdala and prefrontal cortex, they perform unconscious processing of stimuli and emotions. The findings lead to the assumption that mirror neurons perceive consciousness processes such as feelings, needs, expectations in other people and recognize them in oneself, which includes the Theory of Mind. This enables social action, in which one can also put oneself in the roles of others (Bender and Beller 2013).

7.4 Cognition and Emotion Regulation

In addition to these bottom-up systems, there is a *top-down regulation system* located in the cerebral cortex that exercises *cognitive control* by assessing, controlling, and, if necessary, re-evaluating emotions. This system forms the basis of cognitive behavioural therapy. The prefrontal cortex is directly connected with the amygdala and the hypothalamus; it can assess the salience of stimuli and then also make *re-evaluations* of the stimuli, thus exercising *emotion control*. Different regulation systems control different categories of feelings and thus have different effects on a common goal in the prefrontal cortex or the amygdala, thus acting top-down (Kandel et al. 2000; Kandel 2014; Fonagy et al. 2004). The discovery of *re-evaluations* also includes the need to consciously recognize the cause of feelings, thus using cognitive control strategies for emotion control.

7.5 Specific Causes of Fears

This section provides a brief overview of the specific causes of fears.

Example: Dental Fears (according to Kossak and Zehner 2011)

The causes specified using the example of dental fear also apply to all other fears.

Classical Conditioning

- Traumatic experiences during dental treatment (Lindsey and Jackson 1993)
- Intense pain experience in early childhood (Thompson 1999)
- Frequent confrontation with the aversive dental experience
- Increased physiological arousal during treatment, supported by specific smells, often associated with stimulus generalization (Vermetten et al. 2007)

Operant Reinforcement

- Gaining attention and reinforcement through illness

Learning through Anxiety Models

- Anxiety models through parents, siblings (Jöhren et al. 2009)
- Hearing horror stories about dental experiences, etc.

Cognitive Learning Processes

- Subjective assessment of the situation ◄

References

Bender A, Beller S (2013) Die Welt des Denkens—Kognitive Einheit, kulturelle Vielfalt. Huber, Bern

Fonagy P, Gergely G, Jurist EL, Target M (2004) Affektregulierung, Mentalisierung und die Entwicklung des Selbst. Klett-Cotta, Stuttgart

Jöhren HP, Enkling N, Heinen R, Sartory G (2009) Klinischer Erfolg einer verhaltenstherapeutischen Kurzintervention zur Behandlung von Zahnbehandlungsphobie. Deutsche Zahnärztliche Zeitschrift (DZZ) 64(6):377–382

Kandel ER (2014) Das Zeitalter der Erkenntnis. Pantheon, München

Kandel ER, Schwartz JH, Jessell TM (2000) Principles of neural science, 4. Aufl. McGraw Hill Medical, New York

Kim WB, Cho J-H (2017) Encoding of discriminating fear memory by input-specific LTP in the amygdala. Neuron 95(3):1129–1146

Kossak H-C, Zehner G (2011) Hypnose beim Kinderzahnarzt. Verhaltensführung und Kommunikation. Springer, Berlin

Lindsey S, Jackson C (1993) Fear of routine dental treatment in adults: its nature and management. Psychol Health 8:135

Panksepp J (2004) Affective neuroscience: the foundations of human and animal emotions. University Press, Oxford

Pawlow IP (1938) Versuch einer physiologischen Interpretation der Symptomatologie bei der Hysterie. In Pawlow (Hrsg), Zwanzigjährige Erfahrungen mit dem objektiven Studium der höheren Nerventätigkeiten (des Verhaltens) der Tiere, Leningrad

Rizzolatti G, Sinigaglia C (2008) Empathie und Spiegelneurone: Die biologische Basis des Mitgefühls. Suhrkamp, Frankfurt a .M.

Schultz W (2006) Verhaltenstheorien und die Neurophysiologie der Belohnung. Annu Rev Psychol 57:87–115

Schultz W (2007) Behavioral dopamine signals. Trends Neurosci 30(5):203–210

Thompson S (1999) Hypnose bei der Behandlung von Zahnbehandlungsängsten. Hypnose und Kognition 16(1+2):73–90

Vermetten E, Schmahl C, Southwick SM, Bremner JD (2007) Positron tomographic emission study of olfactory induced emotional recall in veterans with and without combat-related posttraumatic stress disorder. Psychopharmacol Bull 40:8–30

Part II
The Combinations of Methods—Theory and Practice of Hypnosis and Behavior Therapy

Behavioral Therapy—Methods
After defining behavioral therapy and the behavior analysis derived from it, its therapy goals are presented, which lead to self-control conviction.

Here too, the individual methods of behavioral therapy (VT) are only very briefly presented and in the aspects significant for the brief therapy presented here.

The Method Combinations
The focus is on the combination of hypnosis and modern cognitive-behavioral therapy with its practical applications.

Autobiography
In a historical overview, the development of the method combination is presented. It is, so to speak, a part of the author's autobiography, his life story of hypnosis.

Life is,
what our thinking
makes of it.
(Marcus Aurelius)

Behavior Therapy—Methods

8

Contents

H.-C. Kossak, *Cognitive-behavioral Psychotherapy for Anxiety*,
https://doi.org/10.1007/978-3-662-69099-4_8

8.1 Basic Requirements

Behavioural therapy is an extremely comprehensive and constantly evolving field of science. For our purposes, we will limit ourselves to its basic principles and assumptions.

8.1.1 Definition of Behavioural Therapy

The term *behavioural therapy* encompasses various therapeutic methods that are oriented towards learning theories. These methods are used to build, reduce, and modify behaviours, including cognitive, emotional, and physical reactions (Schulte 1999, p. 45).

Behavioural therapy pragmatically incorporates methods from other schools of thought, based on the respective need for intervention. This approach was suggested by Lazarus (1973) as *methodological eclecticism*.

Delineation

Unlike other psychotherapy methods, behavioural therapy does not work with constructs such as “personality”, “repression”, or “unconscious”. Instead, it deals with visible and invisible behaviours such as emotions, thoughts, imaginations, and their changes.

8.1.2 Behavioural Analysis—Conditioning Models of Behaviour

The aforementioned models of operant human learning may seem relatively simple. However, they do not exist in isolation, but have developed through certain factors within or outside the individual. Therefore, it is necessary to precisely explore the current state. This is referred to as horizontal or situational behaviour analysis. Additionally, the genesis, or the vertical or contextual behaviour analysis of the learning history, is required.

This includes the exploration of numerous other determinants of behaviour, first established by Kanfer and Saslow (1969) as Behaviour Equation SORKC, which is part of behaviour analysis (Fig. 8.1). It was later supplemented and modified several times (Batra et al. 2000; Margraf and Schneider 2018; Schulte 1999). For basic orientation, only the original model is reproduced here.

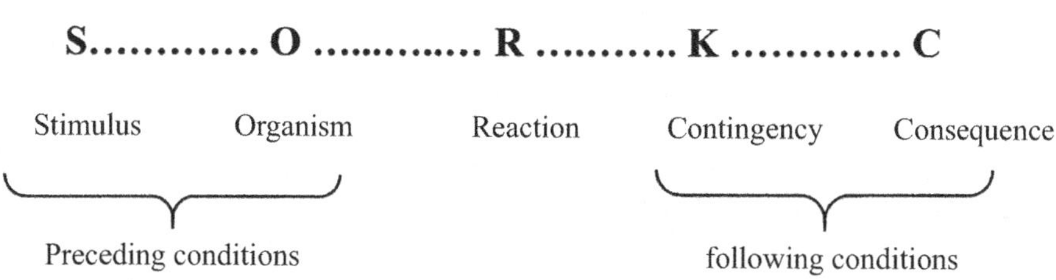

Fig. 8.1 The Behaviour Equation according to Kanfer (1969)
Certain stimuli cause (emotional, motor, cognitive etc.) behaviours (R). Numerous organism variables (O) are effective in this. On this basis, these behaviours are then reinforced (C) by certain circumstances, depending on their contingency (K), i.e. their frequency, regularity and timely effects. S = internal and external stimulus situation that triggers the behaviour in question (R). O = individual biological and learning historical conditions of the person (disease, body, psychosocial environment, medication, drugs etc.). R = reaction to the stimulus (S) after the cognitive, vegetative, affective and motor processing of the organism. K = type of regularity of the consequences (C) following the behaviour. C = the reinforcement (reward, punishment or their withdrawal) that begins as a result of the behaviour

8.1.3 The Diagnostic Interview—Functional Behaviour Analysis

The diagnosis of disturbed or deviant behaviour is carried out through *behaviour analysis.* The aim is, among other things, to explore the triggering causes of the disorders and their further maintaining conditions beyond the identification of a symptom—as in the DSM described - to find triggering causes of the behavior problems and their maintaining conditions. These can lie within the individual itself, e.g. in imaginations or thoughts of fear or in the social or physical environment. Thus, this is a *functional analysis.*

Further goals are to explore resources and deficits, past and present competencies, etc. with the behaviour analysis (e.g. Schaller and Schemmel 2013).

Aspects of Functional Behaviour Analysis (Brief Version of Behaviour Exploration)

- Triggering and maintaining conditions of critical behaviour,
- Genesis and further developments of the problem
- Emotion, cognition, physiology etc. (see the seven-factor scheme, Sect. 3.3.2).
- Self-regulation (e.g. competencies, self-observation, self-reinforcement, self-evaluation),
- Resources—strengths, competencies (past, present)
- Deficits (e.g. cognitive, social)
- Social conditions (e.g. norms, rules)
- Environment (e.g. stressors, profession, reinforcement opportunities)
- Organism (e.g. disease, medication, disability).

From these data and their function among each other, the therapy goals and the indication of certain interventions can then be derived, followed by the differentiated therapy planning of the individual treatment steps.

8.1.4 Indication of a Therapy

The ***indication*** and thus the determination of the goal of one of the many intervention methods starts at various points (Kossak 2015a):

- At the triggering causes and/or maintaining conditions.
- At the clinical diagnoses of the DSM and their criteria.
- At the behaviour problems (target responses), which are most likely to expect changes and their generalization.
- Depending on the disorder or intervention method, sub-goals (e.g. learning a relaxation method) are to be defined, which need to be achieved.

8.1.5 Therapy Planning

In addition to the indication of a method, the planning of the then concrete procedures, the *therapy goals*, takes place. These should—based on the theoretical consideration of the indication—now be designed in such a way that they are applicable after *testing the feasibly real*. That is, they should be promisingly feasible considering the situation, the possibilities and abilities of the client and should be coordinated and discussed with him.

8.1.6 Practice of Behaviour Therapy

Behaviour Therapy (BT) includes a practically oriented form of diagnosis and treatment, which, however, strictly adheres to its basic theories. Due to its variety of treatment forms and its relatively rapid effectiveness, it has quickly gained access to numerous areas of application. VT has primarily developed as a branch of clinical psychology and is now the most common form of therapy in psychosocial care: in outpatient and inpatient psychotherapy, counselling centres, curative health care, prevention and health promotion, rehabilitation, pedagogy, etc.

8.2 Therapy Goals

8.2.1 General Therapy Goals

Regardless of the disorder, problem, or disease, the goal of cognitive behavioural therapy is to treat the causes. If this is not always possible, such as with pain after surgeries, the aim is at least to gain control over life conditions or one's own thoughts and feelings.

8.2.2 Therapy Goals for Anxiety

In the case of anxiety disorders, the primary and evident goal is to be free of fear in certain situations, to behave in a certain way, and to expand one's behavioural scope. However, there can be significant individual differences in the patient's expectations.

Sometimes, to achieve this goal of "freedom from fear," intermediate goals have to be agreed upon, such as recognition by the father (Case 23), acquiring skills (Case 18), or exploring boundaries (Case 21 and 22).

Many people feel at the mercy of their anxiety problem, which can lead to helplessness (Seligman 1983). This makes them believe that they are controlled exclusively by their symptom: either *externally* by life circumstances or other people, or *internally* by their own thoughts or feelings: "The anxiety controls me." Thus, the main therapy goal is often the regaining of autonomy, well-being, self-determination, motivation to perform, and improvement of the behavioural scope, etc.

8.2.3 Individual Goal Agreements

Before the start of therapy, the goals desired by the patient should be discussed to clarify the following:

- Do the patient and therapist have the same goal expectations?
- Are the patient's desired goals realistic?
- Are the ways and methods to achieve these goals realistic?
- Will help from other people be required to achieve the goals?
- Are the ways and goals compatible with other people, situations?
- If necessary, new definitions of the goals and their achievement may have to be made during the course of therapy.

8.2.4 Therapy Goal Self-Control Belief

> **Important**
> The further therapeutic goal of cognitive-behavioural therapy is usually not only to actively achieve or change a behaviour, but also to experience and evaluate this as self-caused and to be convinced of this in the future.

According to attribution theory (Rotter 1966), the success of a therapy depends on whether the individual believes that the change is caused by external factors (other people, events) or by themselves. The experienced location of control *(locus of control)* is then either *external* or *internal* and is later referred to as *control belief* (Reinecker 1999, 2000).

In the further development of these theories, a distinction is made between *social-external control belief* (control by other people) and *fatalistic-external* control belief (control by chance, fate, bad luck, good luck, stars…).

Especially depressive patients or patients with a long history of disorder and suffering passively surrender to their "fate", experience themselves as helpless and at the mercy of others. Or they evaluate that the problem can only be solved by other people, but not by themselves (= external causal attribution).

These *control beliefs* of the patient must also be viewed very differently. Because he may well be convinced that the problem is controllable = solvable, but only by other people or by other events or interventions. These can be insights that are possibly correct and may represent a sub-goal of the treatment as an insight (see Sect. 8.2).

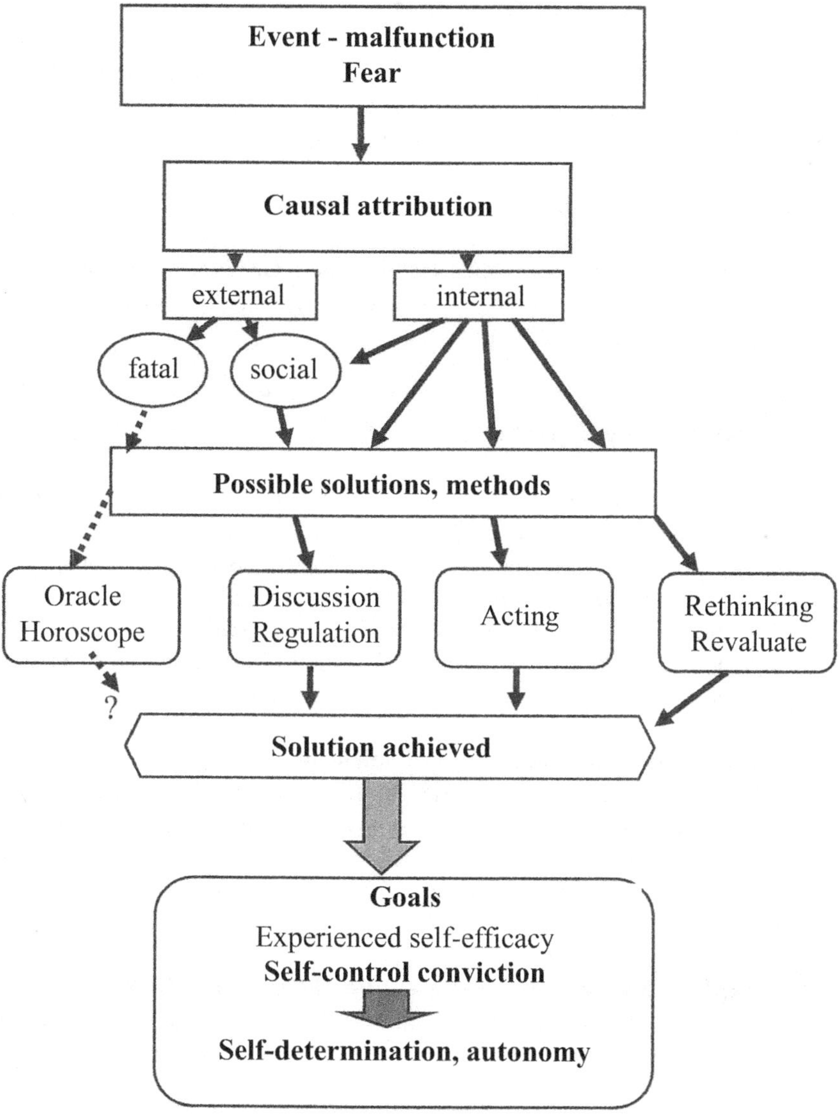

Fig. 8.2 Therapy Goal: Belief in Self-Control
Causal attributions to possible solutions for mental disorders: An event (disorder, fear) is evaluated based on its causation. Subsequently, there are various realistic and unrealistic solution possibilities. Realistic ones include, for example, discussions with social partners, concrete actions, or cognitive restructurings. If one or more of these goals have been achieved by the patient, he experiences his self-efficacy, which fosters his belief in self-control. This results in new or regained self-determination and autonomy, as he is no longer restricted in his (emotional, motor, cognitive) scope and can act freely according to his life plan.

8.2.5 Concrete Goals of Treatment

- The patient should perceive himself as the source of his actions or solutions. This leads to an experience of self-efficacy.
- Self-attribution now includes the understanding that the patient can solve his own problems.
- Result: The patient, with the assistance of therapy, has brought about changes in his attitudes and so on.
- This *experienced self-efficacy* then leads to the *belief in self-control* and ultimately to *expectation of self-efficacy* (see Fig. 8.2)—and thus creates a realistic future perspective (Frank 2017).

8.2.6 Self-efficacy Expectation

- It becomes clear that in numerous mental disorders, the *causal attributions* (internal vs. external) for causing the problem are significant.
- Next, the patient's *control beliefs* are important for solving the problem. The aim is to convince the patient that the problem is controllable.
- Subsequently, it is crucial that the patient *experiences self-efficacyand tests it*.
- Finally, the patients become so convinced of their effectiveness for change that they develop an *expectation of self-efficacy* on which they can rely.

8.2.6.1 Hypnosis and Expectation of Self-efficacy

In hypnosis, self-efficacy can be experienced relatively quickly. Patients are often very surprised at how quickly or easily they can control their fear. Therefore, in short-term therapy, achieving self-efficacy is an intermediate goal until the main goal of *expectation of self-efficacy* and its realization in concrete action is achieved.

8.2.6.2 Explanation from the Perspective of Neuropsychology

The neuropsychological explanation for the rapid change of this fear-based, hitherto resistant to extinction expectation of self-efficacy is probably based on the following:

- Guided by the therapist, the patient experiences that they can achieve positive changes through their cooperation.
- The patient experiences this as a success (C +) and is motivated to continue cooperating in this way.
- This includes the expectation of further successes, thus experiencing anticipation of further rewards (C +).
- These expectations release dopamine or endorphins, which act as happiness hormones and positively reinforce—and the expectation of self-efficacy remains maintained (Schultz 2006, 2007, see Sect. 7.2).

8.3 Classic Therapy Methods—Psychotherapy for Anxiety

Of the multitude of behavioural therapeutic interventions, only the essential ones that have been scientifically tested, successful, and significant for the *short-term therapy* are mentioned here. The focus is on cognitive-behavioural therapy methods, followed by their combination with hypnosis. Their neuropsychological effects can be relatively easily derived from the presentations on the neuropsychology of learning theories (see Chap. 7).

Given the variety of behavioural therapeutic methods, only a brief presentation of treatment methods for fears is provided here in relation to the topic.

8.3.1 Classical Conditioning

The essential methods to mention are:

Avoidance behaviour reduction, prevention. In such cases, the patient is gradually introduced to experience these extended stimuli as harmless through a longer process.

As a therapy, for example, it is suggested to endure the fear-inducing stimuli in slow increase and to become calmer in the process.

8.3.1.1 Fear Confrontation, Exposure

Through confrontation with the triggering stimuli (objects, situations), their harmlessness is slowly recognized. This is facilitated by a gradual approach, combined with relaxation. Depending on the phobia, exposure to the aversive stimulus can be very difficult to achieve therapeutically (anxiety of heights = vertigo, anxiety of flying, tunnel anxiety). The physiological and emotional strain on the patient is quite high in this process.

The goal of exposure treatment is to endure the situation until it is assessed as harmless by the patient

Sometimes, patients even have to be prevented from discontinuing, i.e., from avoidance behavior, must be prevented (response prevention). Self-verbalizations have proven helpful in this form of treatment (Fliegel 1978). These were probably the transition to cognitive restructuring.

Modern confrontation of scenes is now done via 3D data glasses.

The slow habituation to the situation is referred to as *Habituation*.

8.3.1.2 Desensitization

Long known from the history of behavior therapy and hypnosis is the *systematic desensitization* (Wolpe 1961). It works through the graded sequence alternating between relaxation and phobia situation—either in the real situation (= in vivo) or in imagination or hypnosis (= in sensu).

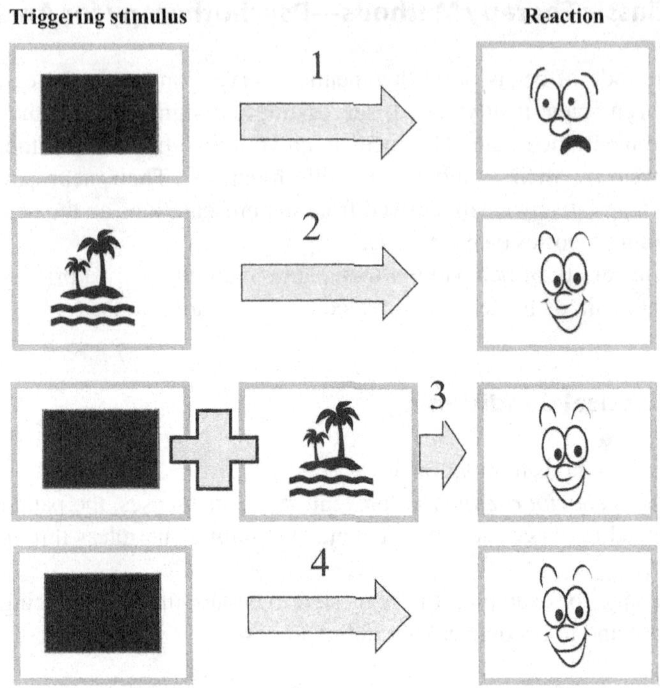

Fig. 8.3 Counterconditioning—Example Fear of the Dark
1 The stimulus darkness (seeing, thinking about it) triggers fear and an increased level of arousal = fear of the dark, 2 The trigger mental and physiological relaxation lowers the arousal level (in the amygdala) as a reaction, 3 If relaxation is performed in real or imagined darkness, the fear is blocked and now calmness sets in in the presence of the former fear trigger (darkness), 4 The stimulus darkness no longer triggers fear, but neutral feelings

8.3.1.3 Counterconditioning

Already in the early stages of learning theories, it was discovered through life experiments that fear behaviors learned through classical conditioning can be reduced if a new behavior (N) incompatible with it is coupled simultaneously with the presence of the triggering stimulus. This reduces the fear (extinction) and is reciprocally inhibited.

▶ Counterconditioning– the Definition

Elimination of a stimulus-response connection by coupling an alternative reaction to the stimulus, where the new reaction has greater strength than the original reaction (Reinecker 1999, p. 164).

The classic example of Jones (1924, 1975)

The child who is afraid of a rabbit is given some chocolate to eat contingent (i.e., simultaneously) with its appearance. The behavior "eating chocolate" (= sweet) is incompatible with the fear, which is thereby reduced. In Sect. 6.1.1, Fig. 6.1 shows the example of conditioning a fear of the dark. Here in Fig. 8.3 it is picked up to illustrate the therapeutic effect of counterconditioning. ◀

8.3.1.4 Stimulus Change

This method can be helpful for both classically conditioned and operantly reinforced fears: The stimulus that has so far triggered the problem behavior is objectively or imaginatively changed and can thereby lose its triggering effect.

8.3.2 Operant Learning—Unlearning—Extinction

We often find relatively simple methods here, which sometimes require the cooperation of other people who have so far had a reinforcing effect and thus maintained the symptom. Only the essentials will be mentioned.

8.3.2.1 Behavior reduction: Discontinuation of operant reinforcement of anxiety

As shown above, fears can also be maintained by positive reinforcements. In these cases, this positive consequence (C +) must be eliminated (Ȼ +).

In our example in Sect. 6.1.2, Fig. 6.3, the mother should not immediately comfort the child as usual. This may sound harsh at first glance and may vary depending on societal norms of upbringing. Therefore, the mother should give affection (reinforcement) when the child can endure the confrontation with the dog a little longer without crying. This way, the child can slowly and gently experience the harmlessness of the dog and will cry less and less until it finally perceives the dog as non-threatening.

8.3.2.2 Shaping Behavior

Here, systematic reinforcements of the desired or alternative behavior are offered, such as the *shaping*, especially in the case of missing competencies. Depending on the number and intensity of the deficits, reinforcements must be made slowly in small steps. Later, possible individual components will be linked *(chaining)*.

8.3.2.3 Changes through contingency management

Here, the patient is enabled to recognize and control the contingencies (= triggering and reinforcing effects) themselves. This brings us to the area of self-control and self-management (see Sects. 6.1.4 and 8.4.3).

8.3.3 Learning by Observation—Learning from a Model—Imitation Learning

In a similar way as fear role models are copied in their motor and emotional behavior by other people, these can be used again after their own fear therapy as models for coping with fear and thereby achieving fearlessness (Bandura 1969). This can be done either through direct observation in everyday life, in the therapy situation, or in imagination, i.e., hypnosis.

8.3.4 Cognitive Methods for Change

Only the essential aspects will be mentioned below.

8.3.4.1 Changing Dyscognitions

In the case of *dysfunctional thoughts*, it is therapeutically helpful to either conduct the *Socratic dialogue* (Beck 1986; Beck et al. 1996) or to make the imaginative/real counter-experience, e.g., through approach.

> **Practical tip**
> In hypnosis, however, no cognitive-intellectual dispute like the Socratic dialogue should be conducted. Hypnosis should rather favor the feelings, evaluations, and pictorial associations associated with the problem (see Sect. 2.5.8.4).

8.3.4.2 Acquiring Self-Efficacy: the central goal of therapy

The concept of self-efficacy from cognitive therapy means that the person is convinced that he can successfully cope with difficult situations and challenges independently. This includes having a *self-efficacy expectation* oneself (Bandura 1977, 1997). This feeling of one's own abilities influences their perception and their performance in many ways (Zimbardo and Gerrig 2018).

8.3.4.3 Reframing—Reinterpretation

The term *reframing* was coined by Watzlawick et al. (1974) and was introduced by Virginia Satir into her systemic family therapy. It was also adopted by hypnotherapy (Satir and Baldwin 1991). In German, it is best described as *Umdeutung* (reframing). A picture frame only shows a section of an overall scene and limits the view, allowing only certain perspectives and viewpoints. Similarly, our view is narrowed by experiences. By leaving this frame of reference, new interpretations and ideas or ways of thinking become possible, such as viewing fear behaviour from a different perspective.

Forms of Reframing (Examples)
Meaning reframing: Find an appropriate meaning for the corresponding experienced problem behaviour, possibly by changing perspectives.

Context reframing: Recognize that the behaviour would be appropriate in a different context.

Case Study 6—Fear of Death

State of Condition
After a major conflict, a young man experienced a circulatory collapse on the highway. While in the hospital, he primarily thinks about death and dying. He interprets the numerous black crows flying past the window as harbingers of death.

Diagnosis
Due to the circulatory collapse and the associated threatening circumstances, real fears (due to heart problems) and irrational fears in the form of dyscognitions have developed.

Prognosis
If the problem situation persists, permanent and even increasing psychosomatic complaints, up to heart rhythm disorders, can be expected.

Therapy
The first step was to change the dyscognitions, possibly then to treat the real fears. The therapist then offered him an imagination scene in hypnosis that it was carnival time for the crows and they were dressing up in a funny way, e.g. one with a red cardboard nose, the other with a turban etc. After a short time, the patient began to laugh at this crazy society, was relaxed and from then on he saw the crows as normal birds that are sometimes dressed up in a crazy way. His fears of death had literally flown away.

Follow-up
Like many of the follow-ups collected, this one was also based on later chance encounters or reports from friends and acquaintances. The therapeutic reduction of fear also lasted for decades here. ◀

8.3.4.4 Priming—Facilitation

Through consciously set or random stimuli (*cues*), existing memory contents are activated and influence the subsequent target stimuli (*targets*) positively or negatively. This activates context information that determines top-down whether the stimulus is recognized and interpreted appropriately (Mayr and Buchner 2007; Tipper 1985).

This mechanism can be effectively used in hypnosis by the therapist using trigger words, imaginations or metaphors that aim to evoke certain memories, feelings or imaginations in turn. M.H. Erickson (1966) called this psychological phenomenon "seeding".

8.3.4.5 Imagination

In the past, imaginations were considered as "unscientific subjective" factors, but it has since been used in numerous forms of therapy, including modern CBT, in many different methods, starting with Wolpe (1961) up to the present (Kirn et al. 2009). Imaginations, or pictorial ideas, are a part of our life, initiating creative processes, showing perspectives and having controlling functions in action regulation, positive and negative affects, recognizing details and their relationships and directing them.

8.3.4.6 Metaphors

The concept of a metaphor (*meta* = beyond, over; *pherein* = bring, carry) involves communicating a linguistic content, concept, impulse, or idea indirectly through an image or a figurative comparison. This addresses different levels of consciousness or the unconscious, which allow indirect access to memories or solutions (Lakoff and Johnson 2018; Gordon 1978). "Older schemas are transferred to newer and more complex facts" (Schmitt and Heidenreich 2020, p. 115), which has also become common in cognitive behavioural therapy (Heidenreich and Michalak 2014); see also Sect. 9.7.

8.4 Cognitive-behavioural therapy in combination with hypnosis—or vice versa

All the aforementioned and the following methods of classical CBT and cognitive behaviour modification can be applied in hypnosis, thereby facilitating numerous changes. In hypnosis, different scenarios and problem situations can be addressed and vividly experienced. This allows the patient to analyse, learn, and test important aspects of self-management (see below) in the protected therapy setting, which then facilitates the implementation in their real problem situation of everyday life.

8.4.1 Commonalities of Hypnosis and Cognitive-behavioural Therapy

The more emotionally oriented methods of hypnosis and the rational methods of cognitive-behavioural therapy have numerous commonalities.

- Relaxation and imagination as important elements.
- Use of cognitive strategies such as reframing, priming, reinforcement.
- The patient is gradually reinforced in their cooperation (shaping).
- The anxious patient is slowly introduced to the anxiety situation (if necessary, habituation).
- Role plays or acting in certain roles with certain actions.

Conclusion: The two methods of hypnosis and cognitive-behavioural therapy complement or even overlap in their practical approaches. They are therefore quickly and effectively applicable on a broad level (compare also Table 2.3).

> **Practical tip**
> In the combination of self-regulation therapy with hypnosis, it is advisable to consider or work on only short and manageable sequences of action in hypnosis (= microteaching). This way, the patient always maintains an overview and is not overwhelmed. The therapist can *immediately* (= contingent) *praise behaviour differentially* (= reinforce).
>
> In addition, the therapist can encourage the patients to observe themselves in this success (their feelings of joy, etc.) and then praise themselves.

8.4.2 A central goal of therapy: Conveying self-efficacy and self-control belief

Self-efficacy and the associated self-efficacy belief can be conveyed or obtained in different ways.

These methods of conveying are also easy to apply in hypnosis:

- **Success experiences**—lead to the strengthening of self-efficacy (experience of mastery).
- **Observation of successful role models**—especially when they are (publicly) rewarded for their behaviour (vicarious experience).
- **Verbal encouragement**—in certain situations, to trust oneself to solve this task (verbal persuasion).
- **Influence of social groups**—depending on support and group experiences, the self-efficacy belief is supported or weakened (social experience).
- **Interpretation of one's own emotions and sensations**—appropriately evaluate physiological and non-verbal signals (sweaty hands, palpitations, tension, fear, etc.) in response to a demand situation (emotional arousal).

8.4.3 Required Skills for Self-Management and Self-Control Belief

8.4.3.1 Self-Observation

The ability to observe one's own behaviour and its situational conditions is crucial. Only with this foundation can the clients later control their behaviour appropriately according to the situation. The patient should direct their attention simultaneously to the execution of the action during self-observation and also to its course (e.g., their behaviour when greeting an attractive person; their thoughts upon seeing an empty wallet; fear, depressive thoughts, suicidal thoughts, temptations).

8.4.3.1.1 Goals of Self-Observation

The goals of differentiation include:

- Learning to distinguish between objective perceptions (dog, person, exam) and subjective/cognitive aspects of behaviour (thought, desires, feeling).
- Observing different aspects or elements of an event.
- Analysing triggers for their behaviour chains.
- Distinguishing critical situations from non-critical ones.
- Making decisions about whether an intervention is necessary.
- Experiencing one's own progress in differentiation, speed, and certainty of their perceptions.

8.4.3.1.2 Positive Side Effects of Self-Observation

Very often, precise self-observation leads the patient to draw conclusions about their behaviour patterns and reaction patterns. This often results in the patient's own steps to change their behaviour (Kanfer et al. 2012).

Hypnosis Methods: Distancing, Decentering

- Observing oneself from the perspective of the "adversary"
- Seeing the whole scene from the perspective of a third person = Decentering (Feffer and Suchotliff 1966).
- Seeing oneself in the situation, but as a neutral hidden observer (*Hidden Observer;* Knox et al. 1974; Hilgard 1989).
- Experiencing oneself within an age regression, e.g., recognizing previous resources or better reaction or evaluation possibilities.

8.4.3.2 Self-Evaluation and Self-Reinforcement

All change processes in life are initiated and stabilized by the constant *evaluation of changes*.

In therapy, the patient learns to perceive their own behaviour and to analyze it in terms of its triggers and reinforcers. In doing so, they will learn to change their personal damaging evaluations (failure, shame, anger, pride, joy).

This is the basis for recognizing in which situations and after which changed behaviours the patient should now differentiate self-reinforcement.

Hypnosis Methods: Self-Reinforcement

- Patients often need to be suggestively pointed out their positive self-evaluation and self-reinforcement.
- The action sequences should be chosen particularly small in hypnosis (= manageable, Microteaching), as especially in hypnosis no cognitive-intellectual exchange should take place, but recognition of feelings and action based on them (see Sect. 2.5.8.4).

8.4.3.3 Self-control—Coping—Decisions

The therapeutic aspects here are:

- *Decision:* Active intervention (change of the external situation) or passive "emotional coping" in the sense of adapting to the external situation.
- Building/using concrete *coping strategies:* "Do I need to change the world, or do I need to change myself?"

We encounter behaviours here that can be conflictual:

- *Resisting* temptations
- *Enduring* aversive situations

It is necessary here to build controlling reactions.

Hypnosis methods: Testingand practicing actions

- In the hypnosis scene, the patient learns to assess his coping possibilities and to implement them as concrete behaviour during and after hypnosis (behaviour rehearsal).
- He can also use small action sequences for practice, or for preparing posthypnotic behaviour in the real situation.
- Especially in temptation situations, alternative behaviours can be practiced in hypnosis, mentally recognised, and then carried out in reality.

8.4.3.4 Self-instruction

Since the patient should be enabled to observe, evaluate, and act appropriately himself, he must learn to internalise the previous instructions of the therapist, i.e., to give himself self-instructions at the individual stages of therapy.

- *Finding definitions:* He must learn to define his actions (including cognitions, emotions, etc.) clearly and precisely.
- *Goals:* He must be able to formulate the behavioural goals and sub-goals positively.

Hypnosis methods: Self-instructionsand post-hypnotic tasks

- The patient learns to give himself the initial instructions/suggestions given by the therapist.
- This also includes completing possible post-hypnotic tasks. He thereby gains action security and better goal orientation.

8.4.3.5 Goal clarification—Goal setting

Together with the patient, his goals, goal expectations, wishes, etc. are clarified (after intensive behavioural analyses have been carried out).

A review must be carried out:

- *Reality content,* being able to achieve this goal—given possibilities, social, financial and personal boundaries.
- *Feasibility:* Can the (realistic) goal be implemented and achieved given the (social, intellectual, material, etc.) boundaries?
- *Social framework:* Do other people need to be involved or "removed" to achieve these goals?

Hypnosis methods: Goal testing

- In different scenes, the patient can experience which of his goals are appropriate and then produce the desired real effects.
- If necessary, the patient must observe from the perspective of third parties that his abilities are limited and need to be redefined.
- At the same time, he can experience that possibly third parties are obstructive, aversive, noxious and others are supportive, benevolent, reinforcing, beneficial.

8.4.3.6 Evaluation of Coping Strategies

This involves the effectiveness assessment of one's actions in reality, asking the question, "Am I doing it right, i.e., effectively?"

Hypnosis Methods: Evaluation

- From the perspective of others (e.g., role model, different perspective), the patient experiences their change and recognizes its effectiveness (*Decentering*).
- For instance, using the "*Video Recorder Method*", the patient experiences their previous behaviours and, in contrast, their newly acquired and effective competencies. With this method, they can view scenes, let them run slower or repeatedly, or observe them.

8.4.3.7 Therapeutic Homework

The patient always receives clearly formulated therapeutic homework. According to their progress and possibilities, it is agreed with them to seek out certain manageable situations and to test or apply them according to the skills currently required (see above: Self-observation, Coping, Self-evaluation etc.).

Hypnosis Methods: Homework, Self-hypnosis

Homework with hypnosis can include:

- Learning and applying a relaxation or rest scene (Anywhere method, see Sect. 11.4).
- Practising self-hypnosis.
- Observing one's own behaviour in self-hypnosis and possibly noting it down for the next therapy session.
- Performing certain tasks in self-hypnosis such as: observation of self-evaluation, self-influence of feelings and/or behaviours.
- In self-hypnosis, giving self-instructions as post-hypnotic tasks to oneself.
- Performing and testing the newly acquired actions or attitudes in the relevant everyday situation.

8.5 Tasks and Basic Settings of the Therapist in Cognitive Behavioural Therapy

Cognitive-behavioural theories and their diverse application methods impose certain requirements on the therapist's working methods. However, these requirements do not significantly differ from those of other therapeutic approaches.

8.5.1 Role of the Therapist

- One of the therapist's tasks is to maintain a dual perspective: to isolate specific behaviours and, despite potential artificial dissection, to appropriately consider the overall context: "Think globally, act locally."
- This also highlights the systemic approach: recognizing "systems" such as friends, partners, family members and their significance (e.g., as cognitive triggers) for the patient (e.g., as reinforcers/punishers).

8.5.2 Relevant Basic Attitudes of the Therapist

- *Active participation of the patient* in actions, problem-solving, self-observation, and decisions is crucial. The therapist's task is to support the patient in such a way that they increasingly initiate independent strategies for problem-solving.
- *Goals are specified in each individual case.* The patient is guided to develop and realize positive and realistic therapy goals. This specification also includes teaching the patient to recognize and differentiate the triggers of their behaviour in themselves and in their environment.
- *Future orientation is important.* The patient should understand their problems against their psychological background and then recognize and plan changes. The patient thus uses the insight into their life for future planning.

8.5.3 Three Aspects of Patient Support

- Learning to control one's own behaviour in specific situations (e.g., reactions in conflict situations) towards personal goals.
- Learning to recognize, influence or possibly prevent specific physiological arousal patterns and emotions (e.g., fear, pain experience).
- Learning to deal more effectively with cognitive (thought, imagined) processes (e.g., self-deprecating thoughts) and to align these cognitive processes with one's own goal ideas.

For further details, see Kanfer et al. (2012).

References

Batra A, Wassmann R, Buchkremer G (2000) Verhaltenstherapie—Grundlagen—Methoden—Anwendungsgebiete. Thieme, Stuttgart

Bandura A (1969) Principles of behavior modification. Holt, Rinehart & Winston, London

Bandura A (1977) Self-efficacy: Towards a unifying theory of behavioral change. Psychol Rev 84:191–215

Bandura A (1997) Self-efficacy: the exercise of conrol. Freeman, New York, W.H

Beck AT, Rusch AJ, Shaw BF, Emery G (1996) Kognitive Therapie der Depression. PVU, Weinheim
Erickson MH (1966) Interspersal hypnotic technique for symptom correction and pain control. Am J Clin Hypn 8:98–209
Feffer M, Suchotliff L (1966) Decentering implications of social interaction. J Pers Soc Psychol 4:415–422
Fliegel S (1978) Zur Wirksamkeit von Selbstverbalisationen bei der Verhaltenstherapie phobischer Ängste. Ruhr-Universität Bochum, Inaugural-Dissertation
Frank R (2017) Therapieziel Wohlbefinden, 2. Aufl. Springer, Berlin
Gordon D (1978) Therapeutic Mataphors. Meta Publications, Cupertino
Heidenreich T, Michalak J (2014) Metaphern in der (Kognitiven) Verhaltenstherapie. Verhaltenstherapie & psychosoziale Praxis 41(4):915–921
Hilgard ER (1989) Eine Neo-Dissoziationstheorie des geteilten Beobachters. Hypnose und Kognition 6(2):3–22
Jones ME (1924) A laboratory study of fear: The case of Peter. Pedagogical Seminary 31:308–315
Jones ME (1975) A 1924 pioneer looks at behavior therapy. J Behav Therapy Exp Psychol 6:181–187
Kanfer FH, Reinecker H, Schmelzer D (2012) Selbstmanagement-Therapie, 5. Aufl. Springer, Berlin
Kanfer FH, Saslow G (1969) Behavioral Analysis: An alternative to diagostic classification. Arch Gen Psychiatry 12(6):529–538
Kirn T, Echelmeyer L, Engberding M (2009) Imagination in der Verhaltenstherapie. Springer, Berlin
Knox VJ, Morgan AH, Hilgard ER (1974) Pain and suffering in ischemia. The paradox of hypnotically suggested anaestesia a contradicted by reports from the „hidden observer". Arch Gen Psychiatry 30:301–316
Kossak H-C (2015a) Indikation und Therapieplanung der Hypnosebehandlung, In: Stavemann HH (Hrsg) Therapie-Tools. Integrative KBT. Beltz, Weinheim, S 545f
Lakoff G, Johnson M, (2018) Leben mit Metaphern. (1980) Metaphors we live by, Carl-Auer, Heidelberg, 9. Aufl., University of Chicago Press Chicago, Il
Lazarus AA (1973) Hypnosis as a faciliator in behavior therapy. Int J Clin Exp Hypn 6:83–89
Margraf, J, Schneider S (Hg, 2018) Lehrbuch der Verhaltenstherapie, Bd 1, 4. überarb Aufl, Springer, Heidelberg
Mayr S, Buchner A (2007) Negatives Priming als Gedächtnisphänomen: Ein Rückblick auf 20 Jahre Negative Priming-Forschung. Zeitschrift für Psychologie. Band 1, 215 (1):35–51.
Reinecker H (1999) Grundlagen verhaltenstherapeutischer Methoden. In: Reinecker H, Borg-Laufs M, Ehlert U, Schulte D, Sorgatz H, Vogel H (Hrsg.) Lehrbuch der Verhaltenstherapie dgvt-Verlag, Tübingen, S 87–146
Reinecker H (2000) Lehrbuch der Verhaltenstherapie. dgvt-Verlag, Tübingen
Rotter JB (1966) Generalized expectancies for internal versus external control of reinforcement. Psychol Monogr 80:1–28
Satir V, Baldwin M (1991) Familientherapie in Aktion, die Konzepte von Virginia Satir in Theorie und Praxis. Junfermann Verlag, Paderborn
Schaller J, Schemmel H (2013) Ressourcen. Ein Hand- und Lesebuch zur psychotherapeutischen Arbeit. 2. Aufl., dgvt-Verlag, Tübingen
Schmitt R, Heidenreich T (2020) Metaphernreflexives Vorgehen in der Psychotherapie. Psychotherapeutenjournal 19(2):114–121
Schulte D (1999) Verhaltenstherapeutische Diagnostik. In: Reinecker H u.a. (Hrsg) Lehrbuch der Verhaltenstherapie, dgvt-Verlag, Tübingen, S 46–85
Schultz W (2006) Verhaltenstheorien und die Neurophysiologie der Belohnung. Annu Rev Psychol 57:87–115
Schultz W (2007) Behavioral dopamine signals. Trends Neurosci 30(5):203–210

Seligman MEP (1983) Helplessness. On depression, development, and death. Freeman, San Francisco, 1975, dt.: Erlernte Hilflosigkeit. 2. Aufl., Urban & Schwarzenberg, München
Tipper SP (1985) The negative priming effect: Inhibitory priming by ignored objects. 37A:571–590
Watzlawick P, Weakland JH, Fisch R (1974) Lösungen. Hans Huber, Bern
Wolpe J (1961) The systematic desensitization treatment of neuroses. J Nerv Ment Dis 112:189
Zimbardo PG, Gerrig RJ (2018) Psychologie., 21. aktual. Aufl., Pearson Studium, München

A Brief History of the Combination of Hypnosis with Behavior Therapy

9

Contents

This brief overview aims to illustrate the shared historical path of hypnosis and behavioural therapy. As I have been involved in this development and continue to work on it, this section serves as a form of autobiography. What is now accepted as standard through the differentiated modern curricula of established hypnosis societies and numerous specialist books on hypnosis and behavioural therapy has been historically developed. Both scientific fields have seen significant development, which required foundational work and enthusiasm.

9.1 Pavlov and Hypnosis

Based on his research findings, Pavlov (1923, 1938) also developed a theory to explain sleep and the similar state of hypnosis. At the core is a neuro-physiological model of inhibition. According to this model, the depth of sleep and hypnosis are regulated by inhibiting and excitating certain centres in the brain responsible for these states. These areas, which Pavlov referred to as *rapport zones*, are reached

H.-C. Kossak, *Cognitive-behavioral Psychotherapy for Anxiety*,
https://doi.org/10.1007/978-3-662-69099-4_9

through verbal suggestions and condition the physiological mechanisms of hypnosis. Words become conditioned stimuli for behaviour or experience in hypnosis.

Building on this, Hull (1933) was able to demonstrate early on that conditioning, i.e., learning processes, are possible in hypnosis—and hypnotic phenomena follow the same laws of learning as, for example, motor actions.

Welch (1947) views hypnosis as abstract conditioning, as a special learning phase for coupling the stimuli is not necessary, since *the mere imagination of relevant stimuli* triggers the corresponding sensation or reaction. He overlooks the fact that the imaginations themselves are usually already conditioned behaviours (such as images, feelings).

9.2 Significance for the Present: Explanation of Hypnosis Induction According to Welch

The therapist gives instructions (= verbal stimuli "*You are looking at the point*"), to which the patient responds with compliance and focuses on the point according to the instruction (= reaction). This in turn is a cue for the therapist to continue formulating like "*Your eyelids are getting heavier*", which in turn is the stimulus for the patient to close their eyes, etc.

This implies that the therapist and patient are in a mutually conditioning control loop until the goal of induction (eye closure, relaxation) is achieved (Welch 1947). Here, operant reinforcement is combined with classical conditioning. Detailed presentations on induction can be found in section 3.1.

9.3 Results From Early Hypnosis Research

Numerous experiments were conducted to scientifically explore the conditioning factors, characteristics, and effects of hypnosis. The simple initial studies of the time yielded findings that encouraged the use of hypnosis—especially in combination with behavioural therapy (Kossak 1991).

The early results include, among others

- Conditioning (learning processes) acquired under hypnosis are more resistant to extinction than without hypnosis (e.g., Hudgins 1933; Barrios 1973).
- The durability of what is learned in hypnosis is thus clearly proven (Smolenskii-Ivanov 1955).
- The generalization of behaviour learned in hypnosis to behaviour outside of hypnosis has been proven (e.g., Welch 1947).

9.4 Early Application of Behaviour Therapy and Hypnosis

Wolberg (1948) was likely the first to deliberately combine behaviour therapy with hypnosis, performing desensitizations and reconditioning under hypnosis.

Wolpe (1961), another founder of BT, popularised Wolberg's method, known as *Systematic Desensitization*. He already implemented the alternating imaginations of the stressful scene and the rest scene in hypnosis.

Salter (1949/1961) should not be forgotten. As a strict opponent of psychoanalysis, which primarily works subjectively and interpretively, he highlighted therapy successes that can be scientifically justified with conditioning in hypnosis.

The renowned journal *International Journal of Clinical and Experimental Hypnosis* dedicated volume 1 (1973) exclusively to the topic of hypnosis and behaviour modification. Many authors use hypnosis images instead of conventional imaginations, resulting in improved relaxation, improved imaginations and facilitated application in difficult patients (Dengrove 1973, 1976). Based on these new findings, Kroger and Fezler (1976) published their standard work *Hypnosis and Behaviour Modification*. They provided wonderful suggestions through plastic hypnosis scenarios like "Shangrila, Robin scene etc.". However, these were—as was the case at the time according to the state of BT—primarily aimed at symptom change.

9.5 Paths to Causal Therapy

The newly emerged BT recognised that conditioning can cause physical and mental illnesses and disorders. Accordingly, the treatment primarily consisted of learning processes and conditioning measures that eliminated these symptoms. Thus, in the books published at that time, it is primarily discussed which symptoms certain conditioning/learning methods are to be used for.

Here we encounter parallels to the earlier hypnosis suggestions, which were also aimed at removing symptoms. The research important for medicine, psychotherapy and hypnosis on the causation of disorders began slowly at these times. Thus, it was also recognised in the aforementioned areas that only causal therapy is meaningful and effective (see Sect. 2.4.5).

Approximately at the same time, behaviour therapy research showed that one can indeed uncover different causes (learning processes) for certain disorders/behaviours. For this purpose, the *functional behaviour analysis* was developed, with which triggers, maintaining conditions etc. could be explored and based on this the behaviour diagnosis could be created, which formed the basis for differentiated therapy planning (Kanfer and Saslow 1969). This was the emergence of causal treatment in behaviour therapy.

Shortly afterwards, T.X. Barber picked up these behaviourist approaches and developed cognitive-behavioural models of hypnosis together with his successors (Barber and Wilson 1972), later cognitive-behavioural theories (Spanos 1991), followed by social-cognitive ones (Kirsch 1992; Kirsch and Lynn 1999).

Meanwhile, we find more and more publications in the 1970s on the combination of hypnosis and BT, but still relatively few compared to other therapy combinations. It is noticeable that predominantly desensitizations and relatively simple conditionings were carried out, which were still anchored in the old tradition of symptom change.

9.6 Autobiography—The Beginning of My Hypnosis Experiences

My professional journey began immediately after I earned my degree in Psychology (with minor subjects in Medicine, Philosophy, and Human Genetics) in 1969 at the Caritas Association's educational counselling centre in Bochum. At that time, there was a significant demand for counselling and therapy for issues such as enuresis, fears, performance disorders, anorexia, and school problems. I promptly began training as a behavioural therapist and psychotherapist. In the early 1970s, the phase of moving away from symptom therapy towards causal therapy of BT began, with the development of various new methods. As one of the first trained behavioural therapists in Germany at that time, I continued to follow the new directions and developments of this emerging behavioural therapy. It was a pioneering period in which notable therapies were developed.

However, I soon noticed that even the highly praised behavioural therapy had its limitations. Therefore, I sought additional methods and, out of curiosity, turned to hypnosis, which I had previously dismissed. I read the diverse findings of T.X. Barber (1969) and the comprehensive textbook by Kroger (1977). The more I read, the more intrigued I became. These scientifically based reports convinced me to start hypnosis training. At that time, we were a group of about twenty people, all fascinated by hypnosis, full of enthusiasm, and dedicated to promoting modern hypnosis in the German-speaking region.

9.7 The Cognitive Turn in Behavioural Therapy

Over the years, it was recognised in behavioural therapy that imaginations, thoughts, emotions, motivation, and attribution are essential determinants of behaviour and play significant roles in causation, maintenance, and therapy. This is referred to as the second wave.

Through the therapeutic application of hypnosis, it had already become self-evident for me to integrate these cognitive aspects into the diagnosis and therapy with BT.

The use of imaginations was then only known in the area of desensitisation. Until then, in contrast to philosophically oriented psychoanalysis, a strictly scientifically based, explainable, and tangible therapy was to be introduced. Imaginations naturally had little place in this context. Metaphors were also considered uncontrollable, scientifically unmeasurable factors.

Case Study 7—*Leg Spasticity*

Clinical Picture and Diagnosis

In the course of these developments of modern hypnosis with indirect approaches and modern causally oriented behavioural therapy, I was asked by a psychiatrist from a clinic to treat a teenager. He had suffered from leg spasticity since birth, which severely limited him. After an orthopaedic operation, he refused to walk and leave his wheelchair. Initially at a loss, I gathered from his exploration that he was afraid of movements that could cause pain.

Therapy
I decided to apply hypnosis, offering him imaginations of pleasant leg movements with indirect suggestions and images. He responded to the hypnosis test SHSS: A with 10 out of 11 points, indicating high hypnotisability, which reassured me as a behavioural therapy specialist with limited hypnosis experience. After just one session, he responded positively and proudly recounted a long, pain-free walk with his parents. This initial success was followed by numerous behavioural therapeutic changes within the family to further promote his independence.

Follow-up
Even decades after the therapy, his gait remained significantly improved and pain-free. ◄

The Integration of Modern Cognitive Behavioural Therapy and Modern Hypnosis
Following my report on this case at a congress, Prof. W. Bongartz, one of the "founding fathers" of modern hypnosis in Germany, asked me to publish the case in the journal *Experimental and Clinical Hypnosis* (Kossak 1983). From that point, I maintained regular communication with him. In the theoretical consideration of this case and the corresponding literature research on hypnosis and behavioural therapy, I discovered that I was likely the first in the German-speaking and also in the international professional literature on hypnosis and behavioural therapy to report a case in which modern hypnosis was successfully combined with modern causally oriented cognitive behavioural therapy. It only became clear to me in retrospect what had previously seemed self-evident: the optimal combination of both methods.

The initial success with this challenging case motivated me to use hypnosis more frequently in the context of behavioural therapy, achieving good results. Accordingly, numerous publications followed in the subsequent decades (see bibliography).

In 1987, Prof. V.A. Gheorghiu invited me to his "First Symposium on Suggestion and Suggestibility". There, I met many of the scientific luminaries of the hypnosis world at the time and was able to learn extensively about hypnosis through direct exchange with them. Among other things, I had the opportunity to speak with the renowned Prof. Hans Jürgen Eysenck, one of the founders of behavioural therapy, who welcomed my combination of BT and hypnosis. In this context, I asked him why he had not published anything about hypnosis recently. He explained that he had worked for some time at the Maudsley Hospital (as director of the psychological department) and had been prohibited from continuing treatment with hypnosis in their Christian-run institution.

I particularly noticed the tolerance of my employer, Caritas director Prelate Josef Ernesti, a Catholic clergyman. He confidently accepted my hypnosis activities and publications. Quite often, I had colleagues from church therapy institutions as participants in my later hypnosis seminars. They frequently asked me to certify the scientific and therapeutic significance of hypnosis and its harmlessness in relation to religion, Christian faith, and application to clients for their employers.

Further Developments

Shortly thereafter, the first edition of my *Textbook Hypnosis* (1989) was created as the first German-language work on modern hypnosis, followed by five revised editions over the now more than 30 years. The invitation to my promotion to *Theory and Practice of the Method Combination of Hypnosis and Cognitive Behavioural Therapy* at the Chair of Cognitive Psychology at the University of Bremen (1992) was then consistent.

The use of imaginations was later named the third wave of CBT. For me, it has been a self-evident method since around 1970.

Since the aforementioned case presentation, about 75 publications, specialist book contributions, and 5 specialist books on hypnosis or BT have followed. I have also given numerous lectures and seminars as a speaker, among other things, on the method combination at different national and international congresses and at training institutes for psychologists, psychotherapists, doctors, and dental associations.

Today, more and more therapists are dealing with the combination of CBT and hypnosis, but the literature on this is still relatively rare, also in the English-speaking world. Alladin (2008) and Chapman (2006), specifically on fears Golden (2006), should be mentioned here.

9.8 Commonalities of Cognitive Behavioural Therapy and Hypnosis

Starting with the then purely pragmatic combination of both methods, numerous commonalities exist from a critical scientific point of view.

What is meant here is not a collection of method combinations of different theories, which can rather lead to a syncretic confusion and is inconsistent. Rather, the method combination is a technical eclecticism in which targeted methods are systematically and comprehensibly selected according to the need for intervention (Lazarus and Beutler 1993).

The following tabular overview illustrates how similar both therapy methods are and sometimes only differ through other, but synonymous technical terms or theoretical classifications. (For better clarity, cross-references to other chapters and literature references, which are already contained there, are deliberately omitted here).

Commonalities of Hypnosis and Cognitive Behavioural Therapy—Rough Overview

- **Requirements for the Therapist**—the relevant factors are identical for both methods.
- **Relaxation**—This is used for calming the physiological system (e.g., Amygdala), thereby reducing thought constriction and expanding thinking and action possibilities, as well as solution possibilities.
- **Imagination**—This refers to vivid inner images or scenes (VAKOG) of selected contents used for diagnostics or as a therapy method.
- **Metaphors**—These are used for indirectly addressing hidden, unconscious thoughts, problem situations, and solutions.
- **Access to unconscious processes**—This can be achieved through therapeutic dialogues, inner images, metaphors, and impulses.
- **Creation and alteration of complex situations**—This involves creating reality-related problem scenes (inner images) that are not or hardly possible in the everyday real therapy setting or are too complex. For example, imagining real scenes in cases of fear of flying, fear of heights, tunnel fear, speech fear, stage fright, exam fear or in very private events such as sexual fears, surgeries, exams.
- **Triggers and maintaining conditions**—These are easier to recognize, analyze in more detail, evaluate and possibly change.
- **Confrontation and approach**—In the imagination, approaches and confrontations of situations, people or objects laden with fear or problems can occur.
- **Systematic reinforcement**—This involves the reinforcement of therapy cooperation and various motor, emotional or cognitive behaviour changes (symptom change).
- **Steering of attention**—Attention can be focused on relevant contents (thoughts, perceptions etc.) or distracted from them (distracted, decentralized, dissociated).
- **Change of perspective**—If necessary, adopt the view from a different perspective (another person) = Decentering—(Hidden observer).
- **Promotion of self-observation**—This involves the self-perception of certain behaviours (actions, thoughts, feelings etc.).
- **Behavioural exercises**—Complex or critical situations can be experienced, played through and tested. This can involve breaking down into individual manageable and controllable behaviour segments and practicing and rehearsing them (Microteaching). Then the correction and reinforcement of the desired behaviour changes and attitudes take place.
- **Promotion of activity**—This involves the promotion of actions, thoughts, solution approaches. It encourages moving away from stagnation towards testing.
- **Resource utilization**—This involves recognizing, applying and testing of known or new resources and thereby behaviour changes.

- **Priming**—Through consciously set stimuli (words, metaphors, stories, feelings, smells etc.) complex or long forgotten (or unconsciously effective) memories of events can be triggered—in hypnosis specifically by means of e.g. age regression.
- **Cognitive restructuring – Reframing**—This involves giving thoughts, feelings etc. a changed, helpful framework or regaining the former accustomed positive one.
- **Improvement of motivation**—This is important in therapy communication and the implementation of worked out solution possibilities.
- **Recognition and acceptance**—This involves the recognition and acceptance **of attitudes and expectations, fears**—of other people or one's own person.
- **Building, experiencing and testing of self-efficacy**—The patient can immediately test his newly acquired emotional or cognitive etc. changes in imagined scenes, to then later use them in the real everyday situation.
- **Action- and Attitude Transfer**—Therapeutic or imagined action exercises create corresponding neuronal changes in the brain. These changes can later be retrieved and applied in real situations as already learned and successfully tested.
- **High Success Rate**, **Effectiveness and Economy** are each characteristic of VT and hypnosis. Together, they create a synergy, thus increasing their effectiveness.

> **Important**
> The diversity of hypnosis methods offers a lot of freedom to design and apply images, scenes, metaphors, etc., thus fostering creativity within therapy.
>
> However, this creativity is only meaningful if it is integrated into a clear scientific therapy concept, rather than serving its own purpose. This is the great advantage of the method combination of hypnosis and cognitive-behavioral therapy.

9.9 Short-term Therapy

As I gained more experience with hypnosis, I became more confident in its application and also learned to recognize my abilities in the procedure. This led to the development of the short-term therapy presented here for fears, first publicly presented and applied at the annual meeting of the SMSH (1989). The therapy successes spontaneously achieved here in demonstrations among professionals confirmed the correctness of my theoretical considerations and their practical implementations. This was supplemented by the numerous positive feedbacks in later professional encounters such as at congresses. This encouraged me to present the method in a more differentiated form in later editions of my book (Kossak 2013). In the meantime, I have successfully carried out the method with many patients and have also received positive feedback from them about the effects and the lasting success of the method after months and years.

References

Alladin A (2008) Cognitive Hypnotherapy. An integrated approach to the treatment of emotional disorders. John Wiley & Sons, Ltd., Chichester

Barber TX, Wilson SC (1972) An experimental evaluation of the new cogitive-behavioral theory and the traditional trance-state theory of „hypnosis“. Ann N Y Acad Sci 296:34–47

Barrios AA (1973) Posthypnotic suggestion as higher order conditioning: A methodological and experimental analysis. Int J Clin Exp Hypn 21(1):32–50

Dengrove E (1973) The use of hypnosis in behavior therapy. Int J Clin Exp Hypn 21(1):13–17

Dengrove E (1976) Hypnosis and behavior therapy. C.C, Thomas, Springfield

Golden WL (2006) Hypnotherapy for anxiety, phobias and psychophysiologigal disorders. In: R.A. Chapman (Hrsg) Hypnosis in Cognitive Behavior Therapy. Springer Publ., New York, S 101–137

Hudgins CV (1933) Conditioning and the voluntary control of the pupillary light reflex. J Gen Psychol 8:3–51

Hull CJ (1933) Hypnosis and suggestibility: an experimental approach. Appleton Century Crofts, New York

Kanfer FH, Saslow G (1969) Behavioral diagnosis. In: Franks CM (Hrsg) Behavior therapy: Appraisal and status. McGraw-Hill, New York, S 417–444

Kirsch I, Lynn SJ (1999) Hypnotic involuntariness and the automaticy of everyday life. In: Kirsch I, Capafons A, Cardena-Buelna E, Amigó S (Hrsg) Clinical hypnosis and self-regulation: Cognitive-behavioral perspective. American Psychological Association, Washington, S 49–72

Kirsch I (1992). The social learning theory of hypnosis. In: Bongartz W (Hrsg) Hypnosis, 175 years after Mesmer; recent developments in theory and application. Universitätsverlag Konstanz, Konstanz, S 173–186

Kossak H-C (1983) Integration der Hypnose in das Konzept der Verhaltenstherapie. Experimentelle und Klinische Hypnose 1:45–56

Kossak H-C (1991) Hypnose und Verhaltenstherapie: Ein kurzer Rückblick. In: Peter B, Kraiker C, Revenstorf D (Hrsg) Hypnose und Verhaltenstherapie. Huber, Bern, S 40–45

Kossak H-C (2013) Hypnose. Ein Lehrbuch für Psychotherapeuten und Ärzte, 5. überarb. Aufl., Beltz, Weinheim

Kroger WS, Fezler WD (1976) Hypnosis and behavior modification: imagery conditioning. Lippincott, Philadelphia

Kroger WS (1977) Clinical and experimental hypnosis in medicine, dentistry and psychology. Lippincott, Philadelphia

Lazarus AA, Beutler LE (1993) On technical eclecticism. J Couns Dev 71:381

Pawlow IP (1923) The identity of inhibition with sleep and hypnosis. Sci Monogr 17:603–608

Pawlow IP (1938) Versuch einer physiologischen Interpretation der Symptomatologie bei der Hysterie. In Pawlow IP (Hrsg) Zwanzigjährige Erfahrungen mit dem objektiven Studium der höheren Nerventätigkeiten (des Verhaltens) der Tiere. Leningrad

Salter A (1949/1961) Conditioned reflex therapy. Capricorn, New York

Smolenskii-Ivanoy AG (1955) Works of the institute of higher nervous activity. Pathophysiological series. Vol. l. The Academy of Sciences of the U.S.S.R., Moscow

Spanos NP (1991) A sociocognitive approach to hypnosis. In: Lynch SJ, Rhue JW (Hrsg) Theories of hypnosis: current models and perspectives. Guilford Press, New York, S 324–361

Welch LA (1947) A behavioristic explanation of the mechanism of suggestion and hypnosis. J Abnorm Soc Psychol 42:359–364

Wolberg LR (1948) Medical Hypnosis (2 Vols.) Grune & Stratton, NewYork

Part III
The Practice—The Case Seminar

After the theoretical and practical fundamentals, now follows the purely practical application.

Description of the Method
The method is presented in detail and in small learning steps, and is very practical in all steps and details.

Case Presentations
Out of a total of 27 case presentations, 16 cases are now documented in great detail: With medical history, considerations for diagnostics and therapy planning, up to the implementation of therapy with subsequent discussion. The inserted study questions allow for interactive learning. With increasing levels of difficulty in diagnostics and therapy requirements, we reach the limits of the method.

The highlight is the transcription of the video recording of a therapy session.

Effectiveness, Limits, Contraindications, Effectiveness
In conclusion, the effectiveness and versatility of the method are summarized, followed by considerations of its limits and possible contraindications.

I must be willing,
to give up what I am,
to become,
what I can be.
(Albert Einstein)

10 The Application of the Method

Contents

After all the necessary introductions and theories on hypnosis, anxiety, and CBT, we now move to the practical part, the application of the method of cognitive-behavioral hypnosis short therapy. However, this is only possible with prior knowledge, as a short form presupposes the complex knowledge from which the essence of the short form has been abstracted.

Now, there are concrete instructions and direct explanations for the individual treatment steps. This relatively large number may initially seem confusing and perhaps even superfluous. However, since the method is very complex overall, it is divided into individual manageable treatment steps.

H.-C. Kossak, *Cognitive-behavioral Psychotherapy for Anxiety*,
https://doi.org/10.1007/978-3-662-69099-4_10

These steps arise, among other things, from the underlying theoretical requirements.

Accordingly, the contents and procedures of the individual steps or methods are each explained in detail. This makes them quickly understandable and then easier to implement into concrete therapeutic action. The case presentations then show the real procedures. The two transcripts of a therapy session, in particular, illustrate the method vividly.

10.1 The Indication of the Cognitive-Behavioral Hypnosis Short Form

The application area of the intensive short therapy presented here primarily refers to "classical" fears and phobias (ICD-10 F 40.x) and other anxiety disorders (ICD-10 F41.x), including panic attacks (see Chap. 4).

It has also been successful in achieving lasting results for smoking cessation.

It is assumed that the method can also be helpful in temptation situations such as diet adherence in obesity. The individual case successes with cognitive-behavioral hypnosis methods in anxiety control in schizophrenia (Maurer 1992; see Sect. 13.3.3) and the control of the frequency of seizures in epilepsy (Heinz 1994; see Sect. 13.3.3) suggest that the intensive short therapy would be applicable here too.

10.2 Requirements for the Therapist

The method is a short therapy that requires experience in long-term therapy of fears to be effective.

The Method Makes the Following Demands on the Therapist

- Training as a doctor, dentist, psychologist, psychotherapist and additional training in hypnosis based on this.
- Sufficient experience in diagnosis, therapy planning and treatment of fears—even without hypnosis.
- Sufficient experience in the application of hypnosis and its combination with known cognitive-behavioral treatment methods.
- This short therapy requires practice and experience with the above methods; therefore, more than one hour will initially be required for this. It is advisable to use an entire session for the anamnesis, to evaluate it afterwards and to create the therapy plan. In the next session, there is now enough time for the planned and prepared application of the recommended short intervention.
- With sufficient experience, the method will then quickly lead to success, as many therapists and patients report. The treatment will then actually be successful in a session unit of approximately 50 minutes.

10.3 Preparations

In preparation for the therapy session, the seating arrangement of the therapist and patient, as well as their preparatory conversation, are discussed.

10.3.1 Seating Arrangement

For the seating arrangement, a corner placement is recommended. This arrangement prevents the patient and therapist from feeling constantly observed. The proximity should be comfortable, yet close enough for the therapist to touch the patient's shoulder with an outstretched arm and later the left wrist, if the patient consents. If not, the touch of the shoulder and wrist should be omitted, and instead, the verbal instruction for rapid scene change must be correspondingly strict.

The typical distance for therapeutic conversations is about 1–2 m; the recommended seating arrangement here is about 35–40 cm chair distance. This brings the therapist into the area of "intimate distance", possibly exceeding the patient's usual critical distance (Altman 1975; Hall 1966) and may cause discomfort in the patient. This should be addressed.

10.3.2 The Preparatory Conversation

The preparatory conversation serves for introductions, information sharing, and exploration or anamnesis collection, possibly followed by the therapeutic intervention.

The relationship building between the therapist and patient, which is particularly important for hypnosis, begins with the greeting.

10.3.2.1 Information About the Session

As with all therapeutic preparatory conversations, information is given about the course of the planned treatment, its method, duration, frequency of sessions, and the patient's cooperation, etc.

10.3.2.2 Clarification About Hypnosis

If the patient is unfamiliar with hypnosis or has questions or fears, these should be addressed. This fosters the trust relationship and provides the patient with reassurance when they are informed, among other things, that they can interrupt the hypnosis at any time and discuss it with the therapist.

10.3.2.3 Building Expectations About the Effects of Hypnosis

Numerous studies show that the patient's expectation is important for cooperation in hypnosis (e.g. Kirsch et al. 1992). To build these expectations, it helps to present the induction procedure as hypnosis and to use corresponding suggestions of sleep, relaxation, and fatigue. This also requires the expectation of the effect of hypnosis to close the eyes and keep them closed.

10.4 The Exploration of the Patient

It is a given that a "conventional" anamnesis is carried out in the sense of a behavior analysis (see Chap. 8).

10.4.1 Goals of Exploration—Precautions

The exploration should also ensure that the indication of the method applies.

This means that a clear differential diagnosis must be made to exclude other disorders also associated with fear. These are clearly defined in ICD-10 (see above).

In the exploration, the patient is asked for the information that is significant for explaining the symptom, its genesis, and maintenance. In CBT, among other things, the triggering events and the associated coping strategies (see Sect. 4.4.1) are particularly relevant.

The aim is to explore which environmental stimuli the patient perceives, how they organize them, then interpret and evaluate them. It is also important to explore how these stimuli influence their emotional experience and actions. This includes identifying dysfunctional concepts and thinking styles and learning processes.

In addition, it is important to determine what role the patient's own responsibility plays in shaping their life with their own decision-making processes.

Precautions Care should be taken not to raise a high level of fear already during the exploration of the fear scene. This could possibly make subsequent cooperation more difficult or lead to the avoidance of further therapy steps, which the patient fears will increase anxiety. If fear arises, it would be necessary in the sense of the planned treatment (counterconditioning) to ask the patient to endure the fear for a few seconds—and then to praise them for having made a good start.

10.4.2 Resource Exploration—It's Not Just Deficit Orientation

The classic definition of problems, disturbances, diseases, symptoms, and their exploration often takes place via a deficit analysis. Thus, every anamnesis in the clinical field of medicine and psychotherapy is deficit-oriented. This approach allows the problem or symptom to be further narrowed down to formulate a diagnosis. Common diagnostic schemes such as the ICD-10 and DSM5 are designed in this way. Diseases are attributed to the loss or malfunction of certain physiological, anatomical, neurological, or psychological balances. The boundaries to the norm or to the normal are fluid. Resources are helpful abilities, memories, evaluations, thoughts, actions (see Sect. 8.1.3, 8.4.3.1, 9.8).

After a diagnosis has been made, therapy plans can be drawn up to "normalize" these changes through appropriate measures for the benefit of the patient, i.e., to heal. Depending on the disease, the patient's self-healing powers, potentials, or mechanisms are rarely taken into account. The transition to health education and salutogenesis is fluid here.

Especially in the self-management approaches (see Sect. 8.4.3) of behaviour therapy, resource orientation or resource management is important (Kanfer et al. 1996) and includes recognizing and supporting the already existing positive sides and abilities of a patient (Armbruster 2015; Fiedler 2017).

10.4.2.1 Exploration for resource orientation

In the case of physical diseases, the patient can actively participate in their recovery, for example, through gymnastics, diet, consistent medication intake, physiotherapy, etc.

In the field of psychotherapy, these resources include, for example:

- Application of relaxation techniques, e.g., with the everywhere method (see Sect. 11.4)
- Application of helpful thoughts
- Application of regulatory measures such as daily structuring,
- Setting up and adhering to certain exercises and regulations
- Self-instructions to refrain from certain behaviour or to carry it out particularly intensively
- Assistance from partners

Therefore, especially in the anamnesis and in the course of therapy, the exploration of previous or current abilities should be of great importance.

10.4.2.2 Resources Aid Healing

Resources are particularly important for therapy planning, as they are skills or achievements with which the patient has already had positive experiences in managing various problem situations. Therefore, they should be a component in planning and therapy.

Under the influence of their illness, patients often focus their perception and self-assessment on their previous actions and problem-solving abilities, so that they predominantly feel at the mercy of the symptom/problem. They no longer perceive their control as subordinate to their will and influence, but rather feel controlled by, for example, fear, compulsion, depression, pain (see Sect. 8.2.3). This narrows their perception to these symptoms, causing them to perceive or judge other experiences as changed or insignificant. Their life then consists predominantly of this perspective of their symptom view.

Practical Tips for Resource Exploration

- In the anamnesis, available resources should be explored.
- If these are not or no longer available or perceived as such in the present, knowledge of past successes and resources is helpful.
- The direct question about the available resources is often misunderstood. This is because the patient may not be able to relate this question to their experience.
- However, the operationalization of this question is understood as, for example: *"What can/could you do well, what do you trust yourself to do, what is helpful for you, what do you succeed in, which people are helpful for you, etc."*—accordingly also the comparable questions regarding previous abilities.
- Sometimes questions for better memory lead to: *"Have you ever tried something that at least helped a bit with NN? What tricks do you use to achieve/reduce NN, etc.?"* With these questions, useful hints on previous or current resources or attempts at self-control are often achieved (see Sect. 6.1.4.2).

10.5 Diagnosis Creation

As shown in Chap. 8, involves a functional behavior analysis carried out on the triggering and maintaining conditions of the relevant behavior. This also includes the deficits, resources, social conditions, etc.

Their effects and functions are then summarized in such a way that a conditional model results, from which conclusions can then be drawn for the following treatment goals and steps.

10.6 Therapy Planning

The intensive, short-term therapy presented here, a combination of Cognitive Behavioural Therapy (CBT) and hypnosis (CBTH), can be applied in a nearly standardized form, as the individual steps and phases are described below.

However, there may be instances where, despite the therapist's best intentions, the data gathered during exploration necessitates therapeutic approaches different from those outlined here. Some brief suggestions are provided below.

Questions and Considerations for Therapists During Therapy Planning
For beginners in this field, the form "Indication and Therapy Planning of Hypnosis Treatment" (Kossak 2015, p. 545 ff.) can be helpful.

- **Diagnosis**

Has the diagnosis been correctly made, or are further exploratory discussions needed to make additions? Are external data required, for example, through behaviour logs or interviews with other individuals?

- **Limits**

Are there limitations from the patient, the therapy method, or the therapist that could hinder the execution of the planned methods?

- **Is Hypnosis Indicated?**

When planning therapy, consider whether the use of hypnosis is appropriate, or if other cognitive-behavioural methods such as model learning, sole counter-conditioning, or systematic desensitization without hypnosis could be equally effective. In this case, a better time economy might be achieved.

- **Planning of Individual Procedures with Cognitive-Behavioural Methods**

Before including hypnosis in the planning, consider which stimuli, cognitions, and their processing modes require interventions, and which interventions from the cognitive-behavioural or other areas are necessary. Could an intervention without hypnosis be more time-efficient?

- **Planning the Combination of Hypnosis with CBT**

At this point, consider which methods of CBT should be combined with hypnosis. This also includes deciding which hypnosis methods to use.

References

Altman I (1975) The environmental and social behavior. Brooks, Monterey

Armbruster M (2015) Selbermachen! Mit Empowerment aus der Krise. Herder, Freiburg

Fiedler P (2017) Ressourcenorientierte Psychotherapie. In: Frank R (Hrsg) Therapieziel Wohlbefinden, 2. Aufl., Springer, Berlin, S 21–34

Hall ET (1966) The hidden dimension. Doubleday, New York

Heinz A (1994) Hypnose bei einem Patienten mit szenischen Halluzinationen als Aura. Experimentelle und Klinische Hypnose 10(1):73–82

Internationale statistische Klassifikation der Krankheiten und verwandter Gesundheitsprobleme 10. Revision. ICD-10. Dilling H, Mombour W, Schmidt MH (Hrsg) (2019) German Modification, Version 2020. Hogrefe, Göttingen

Kanfer FH, Reinecker H, Schmelzer D (1996) Selbstmanagement-Therapie (2. Überarb. Aufl.) Springer, Berlin

Kirsch I, Mobayed CP, Council JR, Kenny DA (1992) Expert judgement of hypnosis from subjective state reports. J Abnorm Psychol 101:657–662

Kossak H-C (2015) Wichtige Aspekte bei der Hypnose-Induktion und Lernziele des Therapeuten. In: Stavemann HH (Hrsg) Therapie-Tools. Integrative KBT, Beltz, Weinheim, S 547 f.

Maurer J (1992) Anwendung hypnotherapeutischer Techniken bei schizophrenen Patienten. Experimentelle und Klinische Hypnose 8(1):11–21

The Intervention—Phases of Intensive Short-term Therapy

11

Contents

This chapter provides instructions for the practical application of the short therapy method, the combination of cognitive behavioural therapy and hypnosis. The introductory and theoretical presentations in the previous chapters are therefore assumed to be known.

H.-C. Kossak, *Cognitive-behavioral Psychotherapy for Anxiety*,
https://doi.org/10.1007/978-3-662-69099-4_11

Cognitive-behavioural psychotherapy for fears – Short therapy with hypnosis—the practice guide

The four therapy phases

The entire therapy consists of four phases with a total of 19 steps.

- **First therapy phase:** Hypnosis—Introduction—Relaxation—Everywhere method differentiation learning
- **Second therapy phase:** Hypnosis—Counterconditioning—positive suggestions – Self-efficacy
- **Third therapy phase:** Autohypnosis—Adoption of coping strategies—Stabilization
- **Fourth therapy phase:** Hypnosis—Termination—Transfer from therapy to everyday life—Therapeutic homework

Now follow the individual phases in detail with comprehensive explanations and instructions.

First therapy phase: Hypnosis—Introduction – Relaxation—Everywhere method—Differentiation learning: Steps

- 1: Induction
- 2: The rest scene– Relaxation
- 3: Learning the body signals for relaxation
- 4: Learning the everywhere method
- 5: The therapy scene—its triggers—Differentiation learning
- 6: Perception of body signals for relaxation

11.1 Induction

The introduction to induction was already made in Sect. 2.5.3. For our purposes, only the two most commonly used induction methods should be mentioned here.

For deepening and practice purposes, it is recommended: "Important aspects of hypnosis induction and learning objectives of the therapist" (Kossak 2015, p. 547 f.).

Practice of hypnosis induction—a small repetition

In Sect. 9.2 on the history of behavioural therapy in combination with hypnosis (or vice versa), it was shown that the induction is to be seen as a mutual behaviour chain between therapist and patient (Welch 1947). From the social-cognitive perspective, this approach is further confirmed in the present by the therapist giving suggestions (= proposals), observing the patient, and then picking up, confirming, and directing the patient's initially only slightly indicated behaviour, such as eye flickering, in the desired direction through further suggestions. For the patient, this behaviour is perceptible and thus proof of the effect of hypnosis, which he increasingly adopts in the desired direction. It is essential that the therapist builds up expectations to continue behaving as hypnosis typically requires of him (Kirsch and Lynn 1999). Possibly, the patient's expectations also need to be served.

> **Important**
> The therapist, acting as a hypnotist, does not have power over the patient.
>
> Instead, the therapist is reliant on the patient's reactions, to which they must respond immediately in a reinforcing manner (see Sect. 9.2).

Among the numerous induction methods, the two most commonly used are suggested here. The induction process lasts from the beginning of the first instruction to the closing of the eyes, approximately 2–5 minutes.

11.1.1 The Eye Fixation Method/Point Fixation Method

The patient sits comfortably leaning back, with their hands resting on their thighs. On the relatively close wall or on the ceiling, there is a point (a piece of paper).

Typically, the initiation involves a largely stimulus-free environment. This already narrows the patient's concentration to the perception of the therapist's voice.

Instruction: Induction with point fixation
Now, suggestions are given that further deepen this focus of perception.

"You are sitting comfortably ... I would now like you to look at this point on the wall. Please keep your head straight and look at this point. Try to keep your eyes open—without blinking. Yes, great, just keep looking at this point, which can be more or less interesting."

The therapist now observes slight eye redness and reacts contingently to the desired changes.

"Please continue to look at the point ... and notice now ... that your eyes are getting tired ... your eyelids are getting heavier. With each breath, your eyes get more and more tired... You have to exert real strength to keep them open. And with your breathing, you notice how the eyes get even heavier ... until they have finally become so heavy that it takes a lot of strength ...

you just let your eyes close ... when you want ... sooner or later... Great, you have now closed your eyes ... and feel your breathing even more ... the calm rise and fall of your breathing ... it is really soothing and relaxing ... to become more and more relaxed with each breath. You are now completely relaxed and enjoying it. ... Now we switch to your relaxation scene. ..."

11.1.2 The Hand Levitation Method

The hands of the seated patient rest on their thighs. For the initiation of relaxation, very vivid suggestions about the lightness or heaviness of a hand are used. The therapist systematically reinforces the patient's reaction tendencies to this. In this way, one or both hands are experienced by the patient as heavier or lighter. The lighter hand even begins to move upwards. This is then a clear sign for both the therapist and the patient of the effect of the suggestions or the hypnosis.

Instruction: Induction with the hand levitation method

There are also numerous variants for this, of which only one is quoted here.

"*Please close your eyes so that you can concentrate and relax better .... Your hands and arms, your shoulders are completely loose and relaxed. Now I will touch your two hands and lift them slightly.*"

Therapist: takes the patient's corresponding wrists with both hands and lifts them slightly so that they are approximately at the patient's chest level and the hands hang loosely.

"*Now please observe which of the two arms becomes particularly light or particularly heavy, feel your hands and arms and their heaviness or lightness.*"

Therapist: now alternately moves one wrist gently upwards (approx. 10–20 cm) and then the other downwards several times.

"*Now observe how one hand or one arm becomes lighter, lighter and lighter and the other hand with your arm feels heavier and heavier.*"

Therapist: senses the movement tendencies and reinforces them by applying slight hand pressure upwards or downwards. When there is sufficient movement tendency in one hand, they let go of both and give the hand a little nudge in the indicated direction.

"*Ah! You notice how the right hand now lifts lightly and you feel more and more relaxed. The hand has become very light and rises higher ... as if there is an invisible thread attached to it, which gently pulls the hand higher .... And while doing so, you switch off completely, becoming more and more deeply relaxed ...*".

Now the instruction can be given to leave the levitated hand floating as proof of their deep relaxation—or to feel the sinking hand as getting heavier and heavier.

The alternative would be to let the hand float up to the cheek. Followed by the suggestion: *"The hand will touch your cheek soon. As soon as it touches the cheek, it falls down and you will then relax deeply."*

11.2 The Rest Scene—Relaxation

When hypnosis is referred to as a relaxation method (see Sect. 2.4.1), it always implies the rest scene. This is a quiet and relaxing imaginative scene for the patient, where they feel comfortable, enjoying the peace and pleasant impressions.

Planning the rest scene
It is important to obtain precise information about the rest scene, i.e., the relaxation imaginations, during the exploration. These should be quickly and vividly retrievable later. The speaking pace depends on the time the patient needs to imagine the picture or scenes. The rest scene therefore takes about 5–10 minutes. With several sessions and home exercises with self-hypnosis, the rest scene with its relaxation effects is established within 1–2 minutes.

Instruction: Rest scene —Green Meadow
"Now imagine a meadow on a beautiful summer day. The sun is shining and it is nice and warm. You are now standing on a beautiful green meadow, seeing the grass and even a few flowers. The sun is shining warmly.

You feel the warm sun rays pleasantly warm on your face. A light wind is blowing, the leaves of a nearby tree rustle slightly. You feel this pleasant slightly cool wind refreshing on your face. Maybe you even hear a bird chirping in the nearby tree, and you look around. The meadow is on a slight hill and you can look far into the country, down into the valley with fields and some houses. They are small and far away, and a river flows there quietly and leisurely. While you comfortably observe all this, you notice how you become more and more relaxed. You breathe very calmly and relaxed. Your thoughts come and go. You will continue to stay calm. Feel clearly your relaxation on your forehead, in your face, in your relaxed shoulders, in your arms, in your chest, and in your stomach."

Instruction Rest scene —At the Beach

"You have a lot of time and spend some of it at the beach. It is wonderfully warm weather, the sun shines pleasantly warm onto your face, also onto your shoulders, and the rest of your body. You can really snuggle into this pleasant warmth. Every now and then a cooler breeze blows, it is also very pleasant and cozy. You look around, it is a beautiful sandy beach, with light, soft sand, the sea is blue and calm. It smells so nice of seawater here. You smell it with every breath, maybe you even taste the salty taste of this sea air on your tongue, try it out. So you walk along the beach, along the water's edge, and clearly feel the water washing around your feet, it is pleasantly cool. Under your toes, you clearly feel how the water tickles with the sand when it drains away. So you continue walking, maybe hearing seagulls calling, possibly seeing a sailing ship with full sails. After some time you might sit down on your towel or directly on the sand. You now feel the pleasant warmth of the sand you are sitting on, and you look out at the sea. The waves come and go, and with each coming and going of the waves you become more relaxed."

Possibly as an addition for further deepening:

"Now you take a handful of sand, it is warm, and you notice the weight of the sand in your hand. While you feel the sand in your hand, it slowly trickles down between your fingers, and you feel the slight tickling of the sand between your fingers. You notice how your hand becomes lighter and lighter, the sand in your hand continues to trickle out and you notice how you relax further and deeper."

11.3 Understanding the *Body Signals* for Relaxation

The following instructions detail how to recognise for relaxation. The patient is advised to place a hand on the part of the body where they can clearly feel the relaxation.

Instruction: Body Signal of Relaxation

"You are already experiencing a pleasant relaxation. Please now place a hand on the part of your body where you feel the relaxation most clearly. ... This could be your stomach ... your gut, your chest, your neck, or your forehead... Please physically perceive your pleasant relaxation at this point... and hold onto this pleasant feeling... for some time."

11.4 Mastering the Everywhere Method

In many stressful situations such as stress or fear, we require relaxation methods to maintain or regain calm, thereby reducing or even completely eliminating stress and fear.

For this, a relaxation method is needed that can be applied immediately and as discreetly as possible, i.e., not recognizable to outsiders, such as during small group performances or public presentations, during exams, etc. This relaxation is learned by the patient through the quiet scene.

In this context, a very easy-to-learn self-control method is extremely helpful. I have named it *"Everywhere Method"* (Kossak 2013), because it can actually be applied everywhere and very discreetly, as it is not perceived by outsiders as a relaxation method or the like.

The often-used mere intentions to relax usually remain stuck at the cognitive level of planning. That is, the purely cognitive level of intentions is often not enough to reliably trigger the required relaxation. This led to the idea of using a *physical trigger* that was discreetly applicable and easy to handle. It was obvious to touch oneself at a point that others would not recognize as therapeutic help. After self-experiments, it then made sense to use the touch of one's own wrist as a trigger for relaxation, etc. Very often in everyday life, we sit or stand and touch our wrist, such as during conversations, while shopping, etc. This wrist touch can therefore be applied discreetly everywhere where stress or fear could occur: in oral exams, during lectures, presentations, case presentations, performances, etc.

11.4.1 The Significance of Joint Touch with the Hand

The physical activity of the hand grip on the wrist and the perception of the touch, etc. are now triggers for relaxation and self-control. The method is highly recommended for maintaining psychohygiene, as it can quickly downregulate to relaxation in "tricky" situations (see above). This learned method of rapid hypnosis works through the conditioned connection hand touch-relaxation.

Esotericists should be informed that touching the wrist does not accidentally or intentionally activate radiations, energy fields, etc., but pure conditionings are intended and effective.

In a longer therapy, the patient is usually taught self-hypnosis and self-control, whereby they train their numerous systems and networks to become more relaxed, especially when symptom-relevant stimuli (events, people, sensations) occur.

11.4.2 Instructions for the Posthypnotic Task (see below)

This simple action in the Everywhere method conditions the body or physiological system and its associated behaviours to become relaxed and free of fear through the hypnosis suggestion (= counterconditioning, see below; see Sect. 8.3.1.3, Fig. 8.3).

Instruction: Everywhere Method

Apply the Everywhere method soon for relaxation
"Whenever you want to relax, touch your (right) hand to your (left) wrist. You then experience your rest scene on the beach, *where it is pleasantly warm and ... (detailed description of the rest scene). You will quickly notice that you are becoming more relaxed, becoming calmer—breathing slower and slower and feeling more and more comfortable. Enjoy this in peace."*

And if you need some peace and relaxation soon, just touch your wrist and you will quickly notice your relaxation and serenity—in your body and in your thoughts."

Apply the Everywhere method as soon as trigger stimuli occur

"You control your relaxation so well that you will also apply it soon when you encounter (the previously fear-inducing stimulus such as seeing a dog, meeting the boss, etc.). You then touch your wrist and notice how you become calm and can handle the situation well .... etc."

11.5 The Therapy Scene and Its Trigger Stimulus—Differentiation Learning

Naming the Problem Scene
In alternation with relaxation, the imagination of the *problem scene* takes place. However, this term should never be used in the instruction to imagine it now, as it always reminds of the problem and can quickly trigger negative imaginations—similar to negation (see Sect. 2.5.1.2).

At the first request, it should be briefly named with a keyword such as in the case of dog fear: *"Now please imagine the scene with the dog; so he is coming towards you ..."* or in the case of fear of visiting the dentist: *"Now please imagine the scene with the dentist. It's a day before your appointment ..."*.

In the following further therapy scenes, it should definitely be named neutrally: *"Now please imagine the* ***other*** *scene again."* This indirectly reduces the memories of negative scene contents. It is thereby relativized in its previous importance.

11.6 Perception of *Body Signals* for Tension

This therapy scene should be triggered by a clear , which will be eliminated in a later step of self-regulation.

Trigger: The Touch of the Shoulder
Such a trigger stimulus should be the touch of the shoulder. It is a "neutral" body part that almost every person can accept. Additionally, this spot is quite far from the later touch of the wrist to initiate relaxation, making it unlikely that the triggers will mix.

Thus, the reaction "imagination of the therapy scene" is initially clearly triggered. A clear verbal instruction as a stimulus to imagine this scene should now be supported by a *noticeable tactile trigger stimulus*. The therapist should touch a spot on the patient's shoulder with noticeable finger pressure and immediately give the instruction to imagine the scene (see above).

As soon as the ends, the therapy scene should begin. The finger pressure and the instruction to do so are given. In the further course, this trigger signal is given until the patient himself initiates the further changes in imagination and therapy image.

Second Therapy Phase: Hypnosis —Positive Suggestions : Steps

- 7: Enduring the Aversive Situation
- 8: Learning to Switch Quickly Between Both Scenes
- 9: Suggestion of the Perceived Positive Change
- 10: Perception of the positive changes of self-efficacy
- 11: Reinforcement self-efficacy and of the body signals
- 12: Repetition Loops—Starting with Step 7

11.7 Enduring the Aversive Situation—Reducing Avoidance Behaviour

The therapist constantly exchanges information with the patient about his feelings, thoughts, etc. during the therapy and relaxation scene. Then, he also notices how and what the patient vividly imagines, when the patient feels tension, excitement, etc.

Instruction: Attention Focusing and Distraction—Reduction of Avoidance Behaviour
Now, the instruction by the therapist follows:

"Please now put a hand on the part of your body where you feel this feeling most clearly. Can you please describe it?" This focus of attention is

now primarily directed at the body's events, and *distracts at least part of the attention* from their previous emotional or cognitive evaluations.

The description of the patients for their feeling of fear (or similar) is often: *"It's such a pressure, discomfort, like a slight burning, restlessness."*

Then follows the therapy instruction:

"Please endure this feeling (tension, fear, pressure) a little longer. You notice that this is possible."

The endurance should last about 30 seconds.

Now the instruction follows:

"Please now take your hand off the spot, just let it sink back down onto your lap."

Please note that the patient should endure this stressful scene for about 30 seconds in order not to reinforce negatively (see Sect. 6.2). This endurance can then already be effective as (see Sect. 8.3.1).

This further prevents avoidance behavior and at the same time causes a habituation to the body feeling.

11.8 Mastering the *Quick Switching* Between Both Scenes

The patient must now learn to switch rapidly between the therapy scene and the relaxation scene, and vice versa.

Rationale for the quick switching

- The objective is for the patient to learn to disengage from the therapy scene and immediately switch, both cognitively and emotionally, to the relaxation scene.
- The more proficient and quicker the patient can switch during therapy, the better the switching will be possible in real-life situations, to immediately interrupt inappropriate thoughts, etc. Thus, the beginning of the behaviour chain "fear" is interrupted, preventing the triggering of subsequent behaviours.
- Through the immediate switching to the relaxation scene, negative thoughts, etc. are blocked, thus inducing counterconditioning. This means: Reduction of negative cognitions (feelings, etc.) by incompatible positive thoughts, feelings, i.e. relaxation.
- The patient initially receives instructions from the therapist for switching, associated with the triggering stimuli of finger touch and wrist touch.
- After a learning phase, the patient will be able to make this switch independently, i.e., regulate his thoughts (feelings, etc.) on his own.
- Since this independent switching is typically mastered relatively quickly, the patient receives clear reinforcement of his behaviour change: interrupt negative thoughts—produce positive thoughts—feel good.

Switching to the relaxation scene – Counterconditioning
Now, the pressure applied by the therapist's finger on the shoulder is immediately stopped, and instead, the therapist grasps the patient's wrist.

Instruction: Switching
Now the instruction follows:

"Please switch now immediately *to your pleasant relaxation scene. Your beautiful rest scene from the green meadow (or beach, etc.). You clearly notice the smell ... etc."*

This guidance will be further reduced in later repetitions of the relaxation scene, so that the patient increasingly assumes control.

As soon as the scene is described by the patient as "optimally relaxed", he is asked: *"Now place your hand on this part of the body that signifies for you relaxation, well-being or security. Feel this pleasant feeling clearly and also hold onto this beautiful feeling. ... We will repeat it more often later. ... What do you feel like ...? Most patients report a pleasant feeling, sometimes associated with words like "free, warm, etc."*

Afterwards: *"Please let your hand sink down again."*

Touching the positive body part
These self-touches of the body parts associated with pleasant and unpleasant feelings focus attention also on the physical and thus associated physiological sensations or relaxation sensations. This facilitates the differentiation learning between the two feelings and likely promotes the intended counterconditioning.

11.9 Perception of Positive Change

The touch on the wrist ends.

Abruptly, the instruction to switch to "the other scene" is given, combined with immediate finger pressure on the shoulder.

Instruction: The Positive Surprise Suggestion
The main part of the treatment consists of a surprise suggestion:

"What has now changed positively for you?"

The suggestion question: *"What has now changed positively?"* is a double-bind (see Sect. 2.5.1) and almost implies: "You have no choice but to report something positive." Accordingly, clients are invariably so surprised that they can spontaneously name positive changes such as: *"I am calmer. My shoulders are lighter. I can look at the dog more calmly. I notice how I do not care. I just think less about it, etc."*

If patients still report no or negative changes like "It hurts here and there", one should persistently ask further: "But a tiny bit of positive change will be found. Let's feel further." Otherwise, we are practically following the patient's cognitive patterns, which are supposed to change. Sometimes one has to insist: *"Well, there will be a little bit of positive."*—Even with major phobias, a minimal change can be detected despite everything.

11.10 Perception of Positive Change as Self-Efficacy

These changes brought about by the positive suggestions are immediately positively reinforced—combined with the hint that the patient was able to do this:

Instruction: Positive Reinforcement
"Great, you managed to be calmer, to think differently, namely: ***I can endure this.*** *This is a success! You have made the start! And later you will continue to notice that you can influence this thought NN (this feeling NN etc.) well yourself."* (Reinforcement of self-efficacy).

Rare Exceptions
Very rarely, patients notice in this first round that they hardly feel anything and are hesitant in this communication. They are probably then unsure about what the question is aiming at, what they should now pay attention to. Usually, it is enough to insist kindly and ask if perhaps something has changed, even if it is little, such as whether they feel less tension (in the shoulder etc.). Now even the hesitant patients can report small changes, which are then differentially reinforced by the therapist.

One should also ask if something has changed at the "problem" body part.

11.11 Reinforcement of Self-Efficacy and Body Signals

Instruction: Reinforcement
"Now please put your hand on the body part where you feel a positive change." Hold on to this feeling of positive change that you have brought about."

If a changed thought (attitude, evaluation) was achieved:

"Yes, great, hold on to this good thought NN (feeling, evaluation): You have brought about NN!"

Here, no intellectual-cognitive dispute should be conducted, but rather an exchange in simple sentences about feelings should take place according to hypnosis (see Sect. 2.5.8.4).

11.12 Repetition Loops

Subsequently, the transition back to the therapy scene is made again, triggered by finger pressure on the shoulder. Steps 7 to 10 are repeated several times.

Instruction: Repetitions
"Please now imagine your scene again ... You are NN ... and now please check again what has continued to change positively! Notice clearly what has changed even more from earlier to now!"

The patient describes their further emotional (cognitive, motivational, etc.) changes and is asked to now perceive how they were able to achieve this. If they hesitate at this point, their sensations described as changes from the previous scene are picked up and offered as a topic. Here too, the patient continues to work with the scenes and the perceived positive changes.

Changes
During the alternating repetitions of therapy scene and relaxation scene, clear positive changes can be observed:

- The therapy scene, which has so far been filled with fear, is increasingly perceived as more neutral.
- Patients usually report on their now experienced changes in their attitudes or evaluations.
- Sometimes they recognize in the reduction of fear that they should perform certain actions such as: simply stand still and negate the dog; talk to the boss; sit in the dental treatment chair and stay calm with the everywhere method; think *"I stay calm ... breathe relaxed ... think of something beautiful etc."* (see Sect. 2.5.1.2 for negation).
- The body part associated with unpleasant feelings becomes smaller and is increasingly experienced as neutral.
- The body part associated with positive feelings is experienced as growing strength and self-confidence.
- Sometimes the negative body part blurs and completely merges into the positive.

When the changes of the aforementioned steps 7 to 10 have been reliably achieved within about 5–8 repetitions, the second therapy phase begins.

The frequency of repetitions depends on the progress of the restructuring. Depending on the patient, the next phase may possibly begin after 3 repetitions. For very large or complex problem situations, several therapy sessions are probably necessary in which individual areas of the problem have to be treated.

Third therapy phase: autohypnosis—Adoption of coping strategies—Stabilization: Steps

- 13: Self-control—Self-regulation
- 14: Self-control of the coping strategy
- 15: Stabilization of self-efficacy

11.13 Self-Control—Self-Regulation

After the external instructions by the therapist, the patient should take over self-control and self-regulation independently and internalize the procedure.

Trigger positive scene yourself

Instruction: Building self-control

The patient is now asked to manage the positive scene themselves:

"Now please switch back to your pleasant scene and touch your own wrist with one hand as I did before. ... You do it just like before: You imagine your relaxation scene for as long as you are well relaxed. When you are completely relaxed, please give me a small finger sign or nod."

Stabilization of self-control

The therapist continues to give the cue for the imagination of the therapy scene through finger pressure on the shoulder—and the suggestive question about the further positive change and its positive reinforcement and the increasingly intense self-control and emotion control of the patient.

This sequence: finger pressure, imagination and positive change of the therapy scene is now repeated about 4-6 times until the patient manages this sequence more and more positively and independently.

11.14 Self-Regulation and Self-Management of Coping Strategies

The patient should now implement the newly learned and successfully experienced therapy steps, or , independently. It is important for the patient to clearly perceive and stabilize their newly acquired self-efficacy.

Instruction: Self-Management

"Please now switch independently between the two scenes. Try to hold each scene for about the same duration as you just practiced with me. Notice how quickly you can switch and how you can bring about more and more positive changes, becoming increasingly confident."

The shoulder touch is now omitted.

11.15 Stabilization of Self-Efficacy

The patient has now directly experienced , realizing that they have achieved self-efficacy through their thoughts, emotions, attitudes, and control of their therapeutic sequences. They have independently worked out these changes and mastered them several times in hypnosis.

As a result, their confidence is high to react appropriately in real-life situations soon.

Fourth Therapy Phase: Hypnosis—Termination—Transfer from Therapy to Everyday Life—Therapeutic Homework: Steps

- 16: Posthypnotic task
- 17: Termination of hypnosis—positive end
- 18: Debriefing
- 19: Therapeutic homework

11.16 Posthypnotic Task

After numerous repetitions and particularly after the patient's repeated and consistent success reports, the *posthypnotic task* follows. In situations that have previously been problematic for the patient (stimuli, triggers), the patient is to immediately apply the learned self-control (see Sect. 3.6).

In this posthypnotic suggestion, the relevant triggers for self-control and emotion-regulating behaviour are precisely formulated to become effectively active.

A New Formulation Algorithm for a Posthypnotic Task (according to Scholz 2006; Scholz et al. 2008)

- The task is derived directly from the patient's hypnosis order. What benefit does the patient want to gain from this hypnosis?—Concrete formulation.
- The therapist encourages the patient to imagine this goal contained in the order.—Imagery, VAKOG.

- The solution—the target behaviour—is condensed into a keyword.—Vividness.
- The solution is linked to external and internal triggering conditions.—If-then formulations.

Subsequent instructions largely follow this formulation algorithm.

Instruction: Posthypnotic Task
"Whenever you think about your problem NN or find yourself in similar situations—or when unpleasant feelings occur as before, you will immediately touch your wrist and switch to your beautiful relaxation scene. You will then immediately switch to relaxation and use your positive thoughts (name)."

Posthypnotic Task using the example of a fear of dogs

*"Always, **when** you see or hear a dog in the future (possibly formulate more vividly), **then** you apply the Everywhere method and relax immediately. You will then **notice** that the sight of the dog has become completely uninteresting to you. You look at him and notice how indifferent a dog has become to you. You notice this very clearly because you are very calm, stand still and feel loose, relaxed. You notice very clearly that you then remain very calm. Also in the future, when you see a dog again, you can let him come close while you stand still. You notice that you stay calm and the dog has become increasingly indifferent to you. ..."* (Fig. 11.1) ◄

Note on this posthypnotic task This formulation assumes that the patient will predominantly encounter well-behaved dogs in the near future, as shown later in case 9. In contrast, case 10 involves a dog that viciously and unguardedly attacked

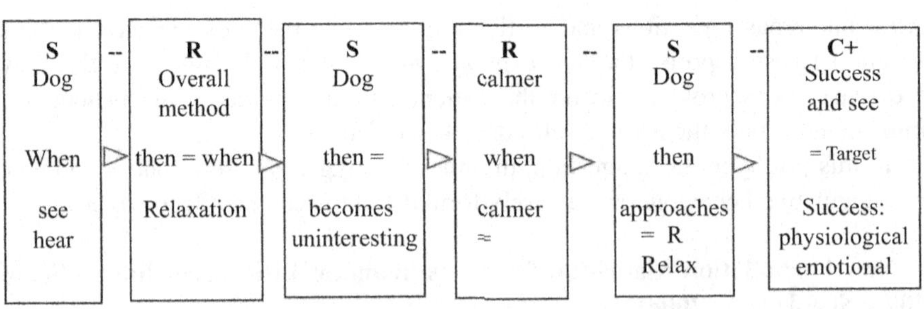

Fig. 11.1 Posthypnotic Task: Stimulus—Reaction—Effects (very simplified representation) The posthypnotic suggestion, *to be relaxed in the future at the sight (seeing) of a dog.* Here the sequence of the individual phases as a sequence of defined stimuli (S) and intermediate reactions (R) to remember the then future desired target behaviour (R) and then execute it

the young patient. Here, the above posthypnotic suggestion is not applicable and must be replaced by other interventions.

11.17 Termination of Hypnosis—Positive Ending

If possible, the hypnosis session should always end on a positive note. This is typically the case, as most patients notice the positive change and feel relieved. However, if the patient reports or exhibits tensions or fears and the session must be terminated, it should conclude with a relaxation scene. This approach ensures the entire session is retrospectively experienced as positive.

If the session ends successfully, the subsequent positive conclusion of the session will further enhance its success.

The termination of hypnosis is typically carried out by counting backwards and reorienting:

Instruction: Termination of Hypnosis
"We can now successfully conclude the processing of the scenes. You were very successful....

"... I will count backwards from 3 to 1 and you will then open your eyes and be completely relaxed, feeling comfortably active. ... 3—You are completely relaxed and very successful ... 2—You are here in this room, on this chair ... 1—You are completely relaxed, feel comfortably active and will open your eyes soon—0—You now open your eyes, are completely relaxed, feel comfortably active. ..."

The therapist remains silent. The patient now has time for *reorientation,* which typically takes about 2–3 minutes. Sometimes, the patient spontaneously starts to share his impressions.

11.18 Debriefing

If questions have arisen on either side, these can now be discussed. This includes the therapist inquiring about the patient's experience of his liberation process. This is followed by further positive reinforcement of his cooperation and the self-control methods and resource utilization he has co-developed.

11.19 Therapeutic Homework

Finally, the application of therapeutic homework and the Everywhere Method in previously critical situations are revisited. For safety, the patient should apply his Everywhere Method at least once a day.

If uncertainties remain or further treatment is needed, the treatment should continue. The entire session should conclude positively, as with the previous phases and steps.

Control Appointments
In any case, further control appointments will be arranged to determine the extent of the changes in everyday life.

References

Kirsch I, Lynn SJ (1999) Hypnotic involuntariness and the automaticy of everyday life. In: Kirsch I, Capafons A, Cardena-Buelna E, Amigó S (Hrsg) Clinical hypnosis and self-regulation: Cognitive-behavioral perspective. American Psychological Association, Washington, S 49–72

Kossak H-C (2013) Hypnose. Ein Lehrbuch für Psychotherapeuten und Ärzte, 5. überarb. Aufl., Beltz, Weinheim

Kossak H-C (2015) Wichtige Aspekte bei der Hypnose-Induktion und Lernziele des Therapeuten. In: Stavemann HH (Hrsg) Therapie-tools. Integrative KBT, Beltz, S 547f

Scholz OB (2006) Hypnotherapie bei chronischen Schmerzerkrankungen. Huber, Bern

Scholz OB, Bleek B, Schlien A (2008) Suggestionen, die erst nach der Hypnose wirken sollen: Präsentation einer Posthypnose-Aufgabe. Zeitschrift für Hypnose und Hypnotherapie 3(1+2):117–126

Welch LA (1947) A behavioristic explanation of the mechanism of suggestion and hypnosis. J Abnorm Soc Psychol 42:359–364

The Practical Case Seminar

12

kognitiv-behavioralen Hypnose-Kurztherapie zur Behandlung von Ängsten—und weiteren Störungen

Contents

12.1 Introduction

In this chapter, case presentations have their broad space for representation. They are presented as concisely, comprehensively, and vividly as possible.

First and foremost, the *hypnosis short intervention* is demonstrated in its wide range of applications and is intended to serve as a model for the readers. These are

H.-C. Kossak, *Cognitive-behavioral Psychotherapy for Anxiety*,
https://doi.org/10.1007/978-3-662-69099-4_12

cases that demonstrate the surprisingly fast and lasting therapeutic successes. They encouraged me to further develop, refine, and compress this form of therapy.

In this part, real cases from my treatment activity with different anxiety disorders and treatment methods are presented.

In case 8 and case 19, there is even a transcript of a real therapy session that was recorded during the therapy. This allows the reader to virtually experience the session with all its details live.

12.2 About the Case Presentations and Case Discussions

Through the case presentation, the reader is involved in the considerations for diagnosis, therapy planning, and therapy implementation. He should be able to understand the author's considerations in order to derive suggestions for his future cases from them.

Study questions

Therefore, particular emphasis is placed on the *study questions* e.g., on diagnosis or therapy planning. These should be answered as soon as possible, as their solutions or answers are given as feedback immediately afterwards. Some of this may seem self-evident to advanced learners; this will help them to get to grips with the method more quickly.

The study questions here refer less to the precise classification according to the ICD-10, but rather to the behavioral analysis of the disorder, i.e., its triggering and maintaining conditions (reinforcements etc.).

The selection of cases

Such demonstration cases should also be very realistic and correspond to everyday therapy. For this purpose, the selection was made not only of simple or particularly well-progressing cases, but also those that involve possible difficulties in diagnosis, therapy planning, or therapy implementation, or even show their limits. Sometimes, difficult or seemingly unsolvable cases or wrong decisions in planning and treatment provide more impulses than particularly smooth cases.

We start with the verbatim transcript of case 8 (Sect. 12.3.1). Its implementation is easy to understand, as here the classic sequence of the 19 therapy steps was possible.

> For a better overview of the 19 steps of the therapy, these are compiled again in Table 12.1. This should facilitate the comparison of the text phases with the therapy steps in the individual cases—and support the learning process of acquiring this approach.

The following case presentations start with simple diagnoses and treatments, until more complicated considerations and procedures are required, until we also reach

Table 12.1 Cognitive-behavioral psychotherapy of fears—short therapy with hypnosis

- The practical guide -

Overview of the individual therapy phases

The entire therapy comprises four phases with a total of 19 steps

---

First therapy phase

Hypnosis - Introduction - Relaxation - Differentiation learning

1. The induction
   Hypnosis induction practice - a short review The eye fixation method/point fixation method Induction with the hand elevation method
2. The resting scene - relaxation
3. Learning the body signals for relaxation
4. Learning the Everywhere method
5. The therapy scene - its triggers - differentiation learning
6. Perception of *body signals* for tension

Second therapy phase

Hypnosis - counter-conditioning - positive suggestions - self-efficacy

7. Enduring the aversive situation - reducing avoidance behavior
8. Learning to switch quickly between the two scenes - counter-conditioning
9. Suggestion of the perceived positive change
10. Perception of positive change as self-efficacy
11. Reinforcement of self-efficacy and body signals
12. Repetition loops

Third therapy phase

Autohypnosis - Adoption of coping strategies - Stabilization

13. Self-control - self-regulation
14. Self-control of coping strategies
15. Stabilization of self-efficacy

Fourth therapy phase

Hypnosis - Termination - Transfer to everyday life - Therapeutic homework

16. Post-hypnotic task
17. Ending hypnosis
18. Debriefing
19. Therapeutic homework

---

the limitations of the method. The cases partly contain simple fears or problems caused by simple conditioning.

In case 8, the acute post-traumatic stress disorder is very complex, but its treatment is "classical" in its pure form and was therefore very clear to present. This makes the method of short therapy easy to understand here. The following two cases of dog anxiety (case 9, Sect. 12.3.2, and case 10, Sect. 12.3.3) and anxiety of flying (case 11, Sect. 12.3.4 and case 12, Sect. 12.3.5) illustrate how different the genesis of anxiety can be—and how differently patients deal with them.

This is followed by cases with spider anxiety (case 13, Sect. 12.3.6) and dental fear (case 14, Sect. 12.3.7) with simpler origins.

In the two following cases, these are real future-related fears, such as the fear of preparation errors for a hip operation, which requires more extensive therapy planning (case 15, Sect. 12.3.8). In the case of real fear of injuries, cognitive restructuring is sufficient (case 16, Sect. 12.3.9).

In the next three cases, relatively dramatic fear situations can be observed, such as panic attacks after conflicts (Case 17, Sect. 12.3.10) and after seemingly unrecognized causes (Case 18, Sect. 12.3.11). In the case of the patient with fear of failure, self-doubt, social anxiety, feelings of inferiority (Case 19, Sect. 12.3.12), there is again a verbatim transcript of the entire therapy.

The penultimate two cases were selected because their history required particularly problematic applications; they demonstrate the modification possibilities of the therapy method, such as in the case of a student's exam anxiety as a victim of crime (Case 20, Sect. 12.3.13), uncontrolled aggressions of a student (Case 21, Sect. 12.3.14) and a young woman with aggressions as a result of criminal influences (Case 22, Sect. 12.3.15). Case 22, Sect. 12.3.15, on the other hand, is a special example that despite a planned short-term therapy, a comprehensive exploration of the patients is absolutely necessary in order to then decide on a therapy.

> **Important**
> It should be emphasized here that in many of the cases presented, the treatment directly or indirectly also addresses the partners in their social system. This particularly illustrates that this short form of therapy is by no means only concerned with the symptom, but also takes into account its significance in triggering or maintaining—i.e., their causes—in the therapy. Particularly noteworthy are the cases: 8, 7, 9, 11, 15, 16, 17.

The indicated *follow-up periods* vary in length. Only very rarely are systematic follow-up inquiries possible in ongoing psychotherapy practice. Thus, one is dependent on the free feedback from the patients. As a result, in rare cases, no information can be provided. However, in numerous cases, long periods of questioning resulted, as the patients were very pleased about their reduction in anxiety and the subsequent improvement in their quality of life and wanted to share this with me.

As in the previous chapters, the cases are numbered to make them easier to find when mentioned.

Reminder

In Case 1 (see Sect. 2.5.8.1), it was a case of washing compulsion, in which the nonverbal and incongruent communications were relevant. Case 2 (see Sect. 4.4.3.1) describes the basic schema of a dog phobia, Case 3 (see Sect. 4.4.3.1) complex cognitions in a fear of flying. In Case 4 (see Sect. 4.4.3.1), exam anxiety arises from negative self-evaluation. Case 5 illustrates how a fear of heights (see Sect. 6.1.3) can be acquired and treated through model learning. In Case 6 (see Sect. 8.3.4.3), the cognitive restructuring of the fear-laden crows at the hospital window was spontaneously effective. In Case 7 (see Sect. 9.7), the suggestion of confidence in one's own abilities helps in a very complex fear situation after an operation (all see Sect. 3).

12.3 The Case Presentations

These and the following case presentations naturally follow the basic concept of cognitive-behavioral psychotherapy with hypnosis. Depending on individual requirements, their variations are then used. This should make it clear that despite many uniform methodological guidelines, the individual diagnosis, followed by the individual therapy planning and implementation, is always in the foreground.

> In all cases, organism variables such as diseases or medications were explored. However, since they were not relevant to the anxiety problem in any of the cases here, they were not specifically recorded or mentioned.

12.3.1 Case 8—Posttraumatic Stress Disorder after EyeSurgery

Emergency Consultation

In the emergency consultation, about three hours after returning from an outpatient eye surgery in a clinic, the patient is still as disturbed as her husband previously described, facially frozen, appears shocked, speaks in sentence fragments about her experience. She repeatedly emphasizes that she had such severe pain, the doctor did not respond to her strong complaints and she was not allowed to cry, so as not to wash the medication out of her eye.

Medical History

Mrs. S. (71 years old) had to undergo a cataract operation on her right eye and was accompanied by her husband to the distant clinic. The doctor was aware that the affected eye had been damaged by frequent inflammations and therefore a stronger than usual local anesthesia had to be administered—or alternatively a general anesthesia. Mrs. S. had heard from many acquaintances that this operation was a harmless routine procedure without pain. Before the operation, she was not informed about the possibility of general anesthesia and a local anesthesia was administered in normal dosage without consultation. During the operation, extreme, persistent and almost unbearable pain suddenly occurred in the affected eyeball. Although the surgeon was immediately informed by his patient, he continued to cut undeterred and wordlessly. Even after the operation, Mrs. S. complained about the extreme pain; the surgeon remarked brusquely in passing, "Well, you survived that."

When Mrs. S. was picked up by her husband from the treatment room, she was, according to his impressive description, completely disturbed, very pale, her facial expression sunken and facially frighteningly frozen, changed as one usually only knows as a reaction to disasters.

She quietly and constantly complained about her pain. It was very hard for her that she was not even allowed to cry, as otherwise the medication would be washed out of her eye. She also repeatedly complained in disbelief that she had been taken by surprise, she was completely powerless, delivered, treated as an object.

After about 40 minutes of car ride home, she was still barely responsive, repeatedly and still in disbelief reported about her pain and the rough approach of the surgeon.

The consultation for psychotherapy could take place within the framework of an emergency concept after two hours.

Diagnosis
The diagnosis of an acute stress reaction in the sense of a Post-Traumatic Stress Disorder (PTSD) is obvious here. Since it is an acute situation, typical symptoms such as hypervigilance or sleep disorders cannot yet be observed.

Prognosis
PTSD usually have good chances of recovery if suitable therapy starts quickly. If it lasts longer, a chronic course is possible.

Therapy Planning
The patient was almost helplessly exposed to the traumatizing situation, combined with very strong physically caused eye pain and the mental effort to prevent tear flow despite the pain. This objective fact cannot be changed retrospectively—not even in the subjective experience.

In the immediate emergency therapy, an attempt should be made to stabilize the patient so that she regains her autonomy, her self-determination, which was brutally taken from her by the surgeon.

In the therapeutic positive sense, it is essential that the patient was able to control herself so specifically despite all the severe pain, not to move during the operation and to hold back tears that would have been damaging. This particular strength should be noticed and used as a resource. She should always be encouraged in her efforts to maintain self-efficacy, to hold back her tears, that only she alone could do so well with her strength and without medical help or other assistance. It is known that those affected by PTSD had to experience their helplessness in a shock-like manner, and especially in post-traumatic stress disorders, the probability of persistence and later flashbacks is particularly high (ICD-10).

The time and content staggered therapy goals are then based on this.

Short-term Therapy Goal
For the present, the aim is to reduce the massive fears, the physiological arousal and to achieve that she becomes calmer as soon as possible and can continue her

usual everyday life—preferably without intense memories of the traumatizing experience.

Further methodical considerations are already being made now, but for better overview in the book, they should be inserted at the relevant therapy sections.

Long-term Therapy Goals

Even if these short-term goals aimed at the present are successfully realized, strong anticipatory fears remain, to be subjected to similar procedures and pains in nine months at the necessary operation of the second eye—even if another surgeon would be active.

Therefore, the therapy suggestions should be directed towards the successful self-control during the operation and also towards the retention of autonomy in the present. Since the self-image is also connected with self-evaluations for future actions, impulses are given for this: She should also confidently present her complaint about her mistreatment at the next operation. Thus, she should feel safer, now having a "tool" with which she is armed and can look forward to the second operation (relatively) calmly, experience herself free from fear and stress—as far as such a situation allows. She should then also be able to demand a different type of anesthesia.

Therapy Implementation

The patient is informed about the short therapy, including the basics of hypnosis, which she is already theoretically familiar with.

She is also aware that a relaxation scene is needed. From the suggestions, she chooses the "Green Meadow".

- **Step 1: Induction**

The patient is familiar with relaxation methods from private courses and corresponding institutes. Thus, she can surprisingly quickly engage in the hypnosis induction. Here, the frequently used finger or point fixation is omitted. Because her operated eye is covered and a point fixation would lead to strong eye fatigue or strain. Because that is precisely the cause of the stress problem. Accordingly, indirect suggestions are used to become more and more relaxed. She immediately responds with deep relaxation.

- **Step 2: Relaxation scene—feeling comfortable in relaxation**

The patient is familiar with the use of relaxation images and scenes, which she has so far been able to use effectively and immediately in case of stress etc. Thus, she can experience her relaxation scene "Green Meadow" within a few seconds and visibly engage in it. During this scene, the therapist, as previously announced, touches her wrist as a relaxation signal by lightly grasping it.

- **Step 3: Learning the body signals for relaxation**

T Please now clearly notice your relaxation in nature, on the meadow. You feel very comfortable and relaxed there… You can clearly hear a bird chirping…

P … Yes, nice.

T (Repeats corresponding relaxation suggestions in the sense of VAKOG.) Now please look at which part of the body you feel this pleasant relaxation, the feeling of well-being, particularly intensely. This can be in the face, in the neck, on the chest, the arms, in the stomach or at another place… Please feel the relaxation there and put your hand on it. … Then feel your relaxation very clearly at this place. This is your personal place for feeling good. … Please hold on to this beautiful feeling there, feel it very clearly there … and concentrate on it: this is your place of well-being. … Please hold on to it for a few seconds.

P (Places her right hand flat on her chest.)

- **Step 4: Learning the Everywhere Method**

T (After about 30 seconds). Now I will show you a relaxation method with which you can quickly achieve your important relaxation feeling anywhere. It's very simple. … Now please touch your left wrist with your right hand—where I just touched it. … and you continue to feel your deep pleasant relaxation. And whenever you want to relax in the future, you will remember this and just like now, by grasping your wrist with one hand, you will immediately be relaxed.

(This is of course a post-hypnotic task, to counteract tension with relaxation immediately = counter-conditioning.) Try it out for yourself.

P … Yes, I understand.

- **Step 5: The therapy scene—her trigger stimuli—differentiation learning**

T Now please switch. (Grasps her wrist.)

(*Methodological considerations:* Since the patient is still suffering from her shock situation, the planned imagination of the therapy scene "Events in the OR" should only be realized briefly, i.e. the traumatizing elements (pain, being at the mercy, etc.) are only briefly mentioned; otherwise, it is to be feared that these feelings will revive and a flashback of the situation with all its stressful drama will occur. Rather, her abilities are now emphasized, despite this situation, to exercise so much self-control of her thoughts and feelings so that it did not get worse = resource use.)

T (Touches her shoulder with his finger). The operation was being prepared in the next room. You are now in the operating room. … There you lie on the operating table … the cloth is placed over your face … there is a slit in it. It is placed over the corresponding eye. … The operation begins … and you experience your stabbing pains in the eye?

P (Visibly tenses up.)

- **Step 6: Perception of *body signals* for tension**

T You clearly experience your tension, your pain. Now feel clearly where on your body you notice this the most. It doesn't necessarily have to be just the eye. Place your hand on this part of your body.

P (Places her hand on her chest, appears facially tense.)

- **Step 7: Enduring the aversive situation—reducing avoidance behavior**

T Yes. I know that this is unpleasant, even very unpleasant, to experience it like this. But it is now very important that you please endure this for a few more seconds. Then your body will remember that you are not running away from it, but that **you** can control it. OK?

P Yes.

- **Step 8: Learning to quickly switch between both scenes**

T Please endure this a little longer. It's important. (After about 20 seconds). Very good that you could endure the feeling. That's a great achievement. That's your strength! (Positive reinforcement of cooperation and enduring the aversive situation = stimulus confrontation, while reducing avoidance behavior.)

P (Nods hesitantly.)

T Now please switch (takes finger off her shoulder). Please switch now to your beautiful relaxation meadow (grasps her wrist). You are now back on your beautiful green meadow, ... hear the birds singing, ... smell the green of the meadow. ... Can you feel that?

P Yes.

T What do you like best about it?

P The birdsong.

(The verbal communication with the patient should ensure that she follows the therapist's suggestions in the desired way and that the rapport is maintained. At the same time, he gets verbal feedback about which experiences are particularly conducive to relaxation and should continue to be used. Likewise, the therapist has the information through this communication that the patient continues to follow his suggestions with her imaginations and does not independently imagine unpleasant scenes and thus escalate in her fear—or leaves the therapeutic framework through her imaginations from other areas and thus shows cognitive avoidance behavior.)

T Now please switch back to the other scene (touches her shoulder with his finger):

P Yes ... it's unpleasant.

T Please endure it for a few more seconds. Later it will become less and less unpleasant. ... Great! ... And now please switch back to your pleasant "Green Meadow" (Removes finger from her shoulder, grasps her wrist). You feel how nice it is there on the meadow ... with the birdsong ... and the smells of the flowers (= counterconditioning).

- **Step 9: Suggestion of the perceived positive change**

Positive suggestions

T Now look inside yourself, what has already changed *positively*. Yes, feel inside yourself, what has happened that is *positive*.
P (softly, amazed) … I am calmer. … Not as tense anymore.
T Yes! Very good! Clearly feel this positive change: You are now calmer, more relaxed.

- **Step 10: Perception of positive change as self-efficacy**

T Continue to feel very clearly that something has changed positively. **You** are more relaxed! **You** have achieved this! Through **your** thoughts and feelings! **You** have brought this about **yourself**. **You** have mastered the situation. Do you notice that?
P Yes … I feel better.

- **Step 11: Reinforcement of self-efficacy and body signals**

T **You** have mastered the situation. This is very important: You should realize that **you** can again determine your feelings yourself. Please feel this very clearly: **You** have brought about your relaxation.

- **Step 12: Repetition loops**

The repetition of steps 7 to 11 follows, until the patient reports clearly after four repetitions how relaxed she feels and the surgery scene has become meaningless for her; she can now look at it without feeling tense, anxious, or excited.

- **Step 13: Self-control—Self-regulation**

T What have **you** been able to improve in the situation through *self-control*? **You** have mastered the situation! **You** have gained more and more self-confidence through **your** relaxation and **your** switching in the imagination and can now determine **your** thoughts, ideas, and feelings again **yourself**, self-regulate. It is very important for **you** that **you** get all this back under control yourself. **You** have the strength to maintain **your**self-determination despite this difficult situation." (= Cognitive restructuring, reframing).
P Yes! (Relief is clearly visible in her facial expression, as she can now even recognize her own ability with which she has helped herself.)

(*Methodological notes:* After the patient credibly accepted this, a way had to be found to change her current state of shock. Since she always lived self-confidently and self-determinedly, the perceived and objective loss of autonomy was a very painful experience for her. Therefore, suggestions for the present and future should be made.)

- **Step 14: Self-control of coping strategies**

T Now you have so much experience in the imagination of the scenes and in switching that you can do this yourself: Please now switch between the two scenes independently. Please hold each scene for about as long as you just practiced with me. Always notice how quickly you can switch and how you can bring about more and more positive changes, becoming more and more confident.

(The shoulder touch is now omitted.)
T Please repeat these changes as often as necessary until you feel completely comfortable. For relaxation, touch yourself by grasping your wrist—as before with the Everywhere Method. Please then give me a sign when you feel sufficiently relaxed.
P (Gives her hand signal after four repetitions.)
T Very good. … How do you feel now?
P Good. Very relaxed and calm. Great.

- **Step 15: Stabilization of Self-Efficacy**

T **You** are always very self-determined and have managed to **control your** situation for **yourself** even under these difficult pain conditions. That means, **you** have power. You are experiencing this right now, how **you** have your self-determination, **your** autonomy under control. Feel very clearly the success **you** have achieved. **You** have maintained this autonomy. Notice clearly how **you** can use **your** power and **your** autonomy again. It is **a part of you and will remain so.**

- **Step 16: Posthypnotic Task**

T If you are reminded of this operation by anything in the near future, please switch immediately by applying the Everywhere Method, by touching your wrist and then relaxing and switching off from this scene as you have learned here. You will then be calm and relaxed. The previous ideas or thoughts about it will then be indifferent. Even if the second operation is due in nine months, you will also be relaxed for it and apply the Everywhere Method if necessary. You will see that it will work well.

- **Step 17: Termination of Hypnosis**

The hypnosis is usually withdrawn by counting backwards from three to zero and the suggestion to now feel relaxed and comfortably active.

- **Step 18: Debriefing**

Effects: A clear positive change can already be observed during the intervention, as facial expressions, gestures, and complexion are now back to normal. The patient feels very relieved, liberated, pain-free and emphasizes that she now has her self-confidence and autonomy again. She can now tell other people about her negative experience in an engaged way, but with a certain distance and a feeling of safety.

As the patient now reports, the suggestions of maintained and present self-determination were particularly helpful, so she now feels strong and notices that she is mastering the problem. This is immediately apparent from her more relaxed facial expression and body posture.

- **Step 19: Therapeutic Homework**

Considerations for long-term therapy goals: The autonomy regained through the short intervention should not only be passively perceived by the patient for herself, but also actively lived out. Therefore, she is advised to inform her outpatient referring ophthalmologist about the mistreatment, so that he can communicate this to the surgeon. It is also discussed whether she would like to change the doctor for the second operation. Since the previous doctor is generally known as a good surgeon, she still wants to be treated by him.

Finally, she is advised or recommended to clearly express her opinion to this surgeon *before* the operation of the other eye. As assumed, this thought is additionally relieving for her. She would like to be able to do this soon.

Posthypnotic Task

Since this thought is particularly pleasant for the patient, a final posthypnotic task is given, initiated by a short eye fixation:

T When you go to the NN clinic for the second operation soon, you will be very confident, because you know that you will get everything under control. Especially when you see Dr. NN, you will tell him your opinion about his behavior at that time in a calm, but clear voice. Please imagine this scene now, calm and relaxed. You meet the doctor in the clinic for the preliminary talk and you will tell him your opinion. You can try this out now. What can you tell him?

P "You! That was very inconsiderate of you during the operation; you did not administer the correct dosage of the local anesthetic and caused me great pain. That was not right." (behavior rehearsal).
(The patient is even more relieved after this formulation.)

T Wonderful, super! You did that well! And that's exactly how you will casually tell the surgeon your opinion. You formulated that well.

Follow-up

The conversation a few weeks after the second operation reveals: Nine months after the short therapy, the operation of the left eye took place as planned. The patient was able to appear confident and anxiety-free in the clinic. The surgeon, now informed about the outpatient ophthalmologist on site, even spontaneously apologized for his behavior. At her insistent request, the patient received the necessary general anesthesia.

In the aftermath directly after the operation and according to reports many years later, she remains stable, free of anxiety, and can talk calmly and objectively about the events. She can no longer remember the details of the therapy session at that time and her psychological state at that time. It has become irrelevant and insignificant to her. This may then be the effect of the post-hypnotic task of step 16.

Discussion

The successful and long-lasting effect of the short therapy makes it clear: Success could only be achieved by additionally aiming for *anxiety reduction* and *regaining self-efficacy*. This also included taking into account the future situation during the second operation.

12.3.2 Case 9—Anxiety of Dogs Since Childhood

Exploration

In one of my seminars on intensive short therapy, a dentist, about 40 years old, 1.85 m tall, 90 kg heavy; a robust man, who is expected to have a lot of strength and energy, hesitantly and somewhat reservedly describes his almost "classic" fear of dogs: as soon as he sees a dog, he becomes nervous, anxious, and avoids approaching by waiting until the animal has passed or he crosses to the other side of the street. This anxiety, which is obviously recognizable to everyone, embarrasses him, he is then ashamed of the devaluation by the spectators. He experiences himself as helpless, at the mercy of others, and perceives himself as a weakling, where he is usually quite brave. He suffers from not having found an effective treatment so far.

The fear of dogs has existed since his childhood. He cannot remember any causal triggers of his anxiety of dogs.

Diagnosis

With a high probability, the anxiety is triggered by the visual stimulus "seeing a dog". The fear has so far been maintained by a) his self-attribution and anticipated external attribution "weakling" and b) his constant avoidance behavior (crossing to the other side of the street) negatively reinforced (see Sect. 6.2.1, Fig. 6.5).

Prognosis

As the patient's life story shows, no spontaneous remission occurred, as even positive counter-experiences were not allowed. The therapy will be a suitable intervention against the long-lasting anxiety here.

Study questions

- Create a behavioral analysis of the triggering and maintaining conditions of the problem.
- Should this instruction to look at and fixate on the dog be sufficient for the patient to relax and reduce his fear?
- Should the behavior of the dog and its needs also be taken into account?
- Create a therapy plan.

Therapy planning

Here, a confrontation with the fear is usually indicated, so that it is experienced that the sight of the dog and the dog itself are harmless. In this context, relaxation through the Everywhere Method acts as counterconditioning.

The *induction* works immediately; as a hypnosis expert, he is practiced in it.

Relaxation scene

He can easily realize the "Green Meadow", as well as the problem scenes "I encounter a dog".

The *suggestion of positive change* influences the experiences very quickly: He can calmly look at the dog and observes how it remains calm.

Therapy Implementation

He is now instructed that it will be necessary to endure the sight of the dog in hypnosis. However, some dogs may perceive direct eye contact as a challenge, a call to fight, or a threat. Therefore, he should not fixate them directly with his eyes, but rather look past them "indifferently". This way, he can safely experience that the dog is also indifferent to him.

During the confrontation, he is surprised. He experiences as a positive change how well he can tolerate the proximity and sight of the dog.

After about four *repetitions*, he can take over the scene change himself to his *self-control* and self-efficacy and experience with relief how his fear continues to decrease and he can look at the dog relaxed.

As a *posthypnotic task*, it is necessary to practice the Everywhere Method regularly, about 2–3 times a week, to apply it whenever he sees a dog—he will then remain completely relaxed.

After about 4 more repetitions, he feels relaxed and free of fear.

Follow-up

In the following years, we regularly meet at the Hypnosis Congress and always look forward to having a nice chat in a group of like-minded people. After about 15 years, he takes me aside and reports that he has been completely free of fear since the intervention, unless he encounters a very large dog. Then he feels uncomfortable, but not afraid. I can reassure him, because this experience he probably shares not only with me, but with many people. Now he hesitantly makes almost a "confession", because he had lied during the exploration for the case demonstration, had understated at that time. Because as a big, strong man, he was already afraid of very small dogs and was therefore ashamed.

Discussion

The patient's cooperation was good, the desired therapy effects occurred immediately and lasted at least 15 years. The late "confession" that he, as such a big man, was already afraid of such small dogs, shows how strong his feared external evaluation was when he was supposed to reveal himself in a group at that time. In individual treatment, this *denial* or understatement might not have occurred. However, sometimes anxiety issues can be so burdensome for the patient that he only reports fragments of them to preserve his self-image—or because he fears negative evaluations by the therapist.

On the other hand, the example also shows how quickly a *generalization* of the fear treatment occurred, which immediately referred to all triggers (= dog sizes) and caused normal freedoms in the behavioral scope. At the same time, it becomes clear that trust in the therapist plays a big role in the exploration and treatment.

The study question aims at the fact that sometimes the partners in this (nonverbal) "fear communication" have to be included in the therapy considerations. So the question is: Will these partners (like the dog here) react cooperatively in the sense of the therapy goal? Do they need additional information for this? Does the patient need additional information for this? Do the cooperation partners also have limits that need to be considered?

12.3.3 Case 10—Anxiety of Dogs—Victim of a Dog Attack

Exploration

Jens, 6 years old, enjoys going to first grade elementary school. He has a severe anxiety of dogs and therefore hardly leaves the house anymore, already takes big detours if he should only see a small dog or only suspects a dog, and therefore has to be driven to school by car.

Genesis

A few weeks ago, the family had a picnic on a meadow when a large dog suddenly attacked Jens for no apparent reason and ripped off most of his scalp with a jerk. This severe injury with high blood loss caused a lot of excitement. The operation was successful and left few visible scars.

Study Questions

- Please create a behavioral analysis regarding the development and maintenance of the fear of dogs.
- Design a therapy plan.

Behavioral Analysis

The dog attack results in a classical conditioning of the fear of dogs, followed by the typically associated avoidance behavior, which operantly maintains the fear. This is associated with a strong restriction of the behavioral scope.

Prognosis

In the case of such severe trauma, long-lasting sequelae such as fears are very likely. Since the child was powerless during the attack, this can lead to reduced self-confidence and helplessness in the long term. Treatment with fear reduction will promote the child's psychological development.

Treatment Plan

Fear reduction through counterconditioning or habituation is the first choice here. A corresponding confrontation with a dog can only be a theoretical solution, as it is hardly feasible in practice and can also be a strong burden for Jens. Therefore, therapy in sensu = in hypnosis is appropriate. It is not necessarily to be assumed that this intervention will completely eliminate the fear. Therefore, the coping behavior acquired in hypnosis should be tested in reality on the way to school. The cooperation of the mother as a co-therapist is required for this, to accompany him to school and then gradually reduce her help. Ultimately, Jens should regain his self-confidence and trust in his own competencies. It should be clarified whether he can respond appropriately to short-term therapy at the age of 6. Further consideration should be given to whether he can or should go to school alone immediately after—if he is then free of fear.

Therapy Implementation

Jens is very alert, cooperative; you can have a good conversation with him. Thus, we can at least try whether the application of intensive short-term therapy is possible and helpful at this age.

He responds well to the *child-friendly induction*. (It and the entire communication must be conducted in child-friendly simple language.)

In consultation with him, a visit to a magic forest is chosen as the *relaxation scene*, where there are colorful flowers, friendly animals, etc. (Kossak and Zehner 2011). He also responds spontaneously well to it with relaxation.

In the *therapy scene*, a small dog, which Jens knows as friendly, comes from afar. Jens can look at the dog with relaxation and does not have to show avoidance behavior. After a few repetitions in hypnosis, he can also encounter larger dogs without fear (= desensitization). He is very surprised at how quickly improvements in terms of relaxation occur (after the positive suggestion). To improve his self-control, I advise him never to stare at dogs and to move calmly, etc. We also practice this passing by in hypnosis.

The *post-hypnotic task* is to apply the Everywhere Method immediately when he should see, hear, etc., a dog.

Mother's Consultation

In parallel, the mother is instructed to act in the same sense as a co-therapist in everyday life, e.g., on the way to school, so when a dog appears, to give the usual relaxation instructions, which she does well. After the first session, Jens is almost free of fear, and the mother can now gradually withdraw, allowing Jens to make his way to school independently again, which he was previously able to do well.

Only after about three couple sessions does the mother mention that the offender's dog belongs to a neighbor and is still allowed to run around outside the property unsupervised and without a leash. Jens rightly still feels realistically threatened.

Study Question

- Is the treatment here completed or should further interventions take place? Which do you recommend?

Since the offender's dog can still be threatening, further interventions must now take place. Clear regulations must be demanded from the dog owner (also legally) to protect the child. Since Jens could not be protected during the dog attack (by his father), he may have lost trust in his father as a protector, possibly generally the trust in adults. Therefore, it is important that the father holds the dog owner clearly accountable in the presence of his son.

Conversation with Both Parents

Now it should be the father's task to clearly demand the neighbor to leash the dog according to applicable regulations, otherwise he will take legal action against him. The father is very uncomfortable with this request and wants to avoid it, as the neighbor is also a business friend. However, it is made clear to him that he must conduct this serious conversation clearly, distinctly, and demandingly and in the *presence of his son*. Only in this way can Jens continue to feel actively protected and cared for by his father, which he could not experience before.

Effects

After these interventions, especially after the joint admonition of the neighbor, all family members feel relieved. Jens now feels protected as before and his fears are soon completely eliminated.

Sister with Fear of Dogs

A few weeks later, his sister, who is two years older, is introduced at her request due to her fear of dogs. At the time of the initial anamnesis, she had no fear to complain about. A relatively harmless recent dog experience suddenly reminded her of her brother's accident. It was the flashback of her own shock trauma that had been triggered. She had been able to observe the entire attack scene up close, such as the blood, the excitement, the emergency doctors in action, etc. This can be classified as post-traumatic stress disorder.

Accordingly, short-term hypnotherapy is applied to her. Her trauma-related inner images and evaluations quickly change. However, she needs about three sessions to be sustainably free of fear and self-confident.

Follow-up

Over a subsequent period of one year, the further stability of the children's anxiety-free behavior is confirmed.

Discussion

Here, the classic case of conditioning through trauma is recognizable, which has generalized effects. As it became clear, the intensive method also works in a relatively young child. Self-control methods are not always consistently applied by children. To ensure that complete freedom from fear exists, several sessions were recommended, also to give the mother confidence in the method.

The focus is now on treating the family system with its conditions that maintain fear (see Sect. 6.2). In the treatment, the *role of the father* also became significant. The father should have acted as a protector. However, since he wanted to avoid conflicts with the dog owner, he was thus a very poor model for self-confidence, conflict resolution, and protector of the family. He could only correct this alone by demandingly confronting the dog owner in the presence of his son. Now Jens knew and felt that he also has stability at this level and will continue to get it.

At the same time, the sister's fear shows how covertly fear developments can progress, even initially being denied, until they break out consciously (see Sect. 4.4.1). Even small triggers are then sufficient; sometimes even very subtle stimuli can be enough, which are not perceived as such by the person concerned, but nevertheless "out of the blue" trigger fear (Priming, see Sect. 8.3.4.4).

12.3.4 Case 11—Anxiety of Flying for Many Years

Exploration

The approximately 37-year-old woman, MTA, is afraid of flying. She wants to make a holiday flight to Southern Europe with her husband and her two small children in about 2 weeks. For several weeks now, she has had to think very often about how great her fear of flying is. She does not want to be a model of fear for her children. She generally sees herself as quite self-confident and self-determined, both in her part-time job as an MTA, as well as in her circle of friends and in other groups. She cannot report any traumatizing experiences in her past. Her fear of flying has existed for many years. She only has thoughts of fear, probably due to corresponding reports and documentaries on television.

Study Questions

- Create a behavioral analysis of the triggering and maintaining conditions of the problem.
- Design the individual steps for a therapy.

Behavioral Analysis

A (Trigger: Thoughts of the flight) causes—B (Belief/Dyscognition: Fear is dangerous) causes—C (Consequences: Thought: "I am a negative example for my children."). The upcoming flight date and the sight of the children maintain the thoughts of fear. She feels guilty about being a negative role model for her children (see Sect. 6.1.3).

Prognosis
If the fear persists, the mother could become overprotective towards the children due to her guilt, which is a cognitive avoidance behavior for her guilt. The patient wants to be a positive role model for her children again. Therefore, she has a strong motivation to change, which has a favorable effect on the course of therapy.

Treatment Plan
Since these are cognitively induced anxieties, the patient should experience and judge for herself which thoughts cause her fear. Since numerous events occur as behavioral chains (such as packing suitcases, driving to the airport) up to the flight itself, which can be associated with fear, the patient should also experience these in hypnosis and continue to feel free from fear. Counterconditioning should then take place through relaxation in hypnosis. At the same time, she should experience and practice in hypnosis how she calmly prepares for the trip with the children. She then experiences relaxation, associated with freedom from fear, and can give up her dyscognition.

Treatment Implementation
The *induction* is immediately successful through point fixation.

The *rest scene* "Green Meadow" is well imagined, produces good relaxation.

Therapy Scene
During the *imagination* of the fear scenes and the request to bring about *positive changes*, she notices that she actually has baseless fear fantasies, because an airplane is stable. She can now experience these inner images, which she has recognized as baseless, as neutral after a few repetitions and independently control them with the Everywhere Method (= *self-efficacy*).

Study Question

- How should the therapy session be continued? That is, what methods or suggestions should follow now?

Continuation of the Therapy Session
To support, post-hypnotic tasks should help: Since there are still two weeks to bridge until the departure date, she should use the Everywhere Method for relaxation and maintenance of cognitive restructuring.

The *post-hypnotic tasks* consist of practicing this short therapy method with the Everywhere Method. For this, she will be a calm and self-confident role model, both in the flight preparations and during the flight itself: In individual scenes, she experiences how she calmly packs the suitcases, buckles herself and her children calmly in the airplane, they look out of the window etc. She is also suggested with the task to order a holiday drink for herself and her children and to enjoy it (= counterconditioning). In the meantime, she should implement the hypnosis actions in real actions in the two weeks until departure and also experience her freedom from fear motorically.

Follow-up

A few weeks after returning from the trip, the client reports that she made very relaxed flight preparations, felt overall comfortable during it and enjoyed the flight including the view and drinks—as did her children.

In encounters after several years, she reports: From then on, flying was not only fear-neutral for her in the following years, but positively connotated, no more talk of fear of flying. She even enjoys drinking coffee and looking out during the flight.

Discussion

Here it becomes clear that cognitive elements alone, such as negative reports and the resulting expectations, have caused fear. In this purely cognitive causation, the responsibility for the children can quickly arise (as cognitive control)—as in the aforementioned case. Therefore, it is likely that the fear will now become greater.

So the post-hypnotic suggestions are directed at the patient herself, to be able to be calm—and at the same time at her responsibility towards the children. Since these are strong abstractions, the suggestions now contain concrete and clear instructions for action (packing suitcases, buckling children, etc.), combined with relaxation emotions.

Through this post-hypnotic task, the patient was able to quickly experience how she could very quickly interrupt this chain of apprehensions. Based on the neutral reactions of her children, she could immediately recognize that she was behaving appropriately (= positive reinforcement), and quickly reduce her fears.

12.3.5 Case 12—Anxiety of Flying After Traumatic Flight Experience

Medical History

The client is 20 years old, a commercial employee and student, single. She wants to fly to Turkey with her parents for the holidays in 14 days, but she has a fear of flying.

Origin: When she was 11 years old, she was on a flight back from the USA to Germany with her parents, during which there were severe and probably threatening turbulences. All passengers, like her, were very scared and screamed. Now, after this traumatic experience, she is anxious, but still wants to take the flight—hopefully after successful therapy. Years later, fear arose again on a flight to Mallorca and increased after watching a disaster movie.

Current situation: She believes that she gives up control when she hears noises like beeping in the airplane, so that she then feels helpless. Therefore, she has to sit in an aisle seat so that she can maintain a sense of control, the escape route is clear, and she can always see the stewardess. She had the thought: "*I will now be locked up for four hours.*"

Overall, she is very sensitive when driving a car, cannot tolerate backward travel on the train, often gets up, needs to be able to look out and then have a fixation point so that she does not feel sick. In addition, she has a high sensitivity to noise in trains, buses, airplanes, and boats. She does not have a fear of heights.

Based on her descriptions (and also the assessments of her colleagues), the client can be described as a normally self-confident and generally anxiety-free person. Her acquired fear of flying has not generalized to other areas, but now only reappears when she is actually planning her flight. The previous approx. 6 sessions with a psychologist were unsuccessful; there she was supposed to write down the pros and cons of her fear and did exercises for breath relaxation. The Tavor prescribed by the doctor also did not bring any success.

Study Questions

- Please make a diagnosis in the sense of behavioral analysis.
- Consider a treatment plan.

Behavioral Diagnosis/Behavioral Analysis

Due to a traumatic flight experience, the patient has a conditioned classical flight phobia, which has generalized, as the patient subsequently fears loss of control and claustrophobia. In addition to the physiological components of fear, cognitions such as negative expectations and dyscognitions, possibly also helplessness, come into play.

Prognosis

It is questionable whether spontaneous remissions occur after such a traumatic experience. The patient has a strong motivation to change, which is very favorable for successful therapy. Since she was then at the mercy of the situation, which caused generalized dyscognitions, short-term therapy with cognitive restructuring seems to have a favorable prognosis.

Treatment Plan

With the existing fears of loss of control, the patient should regain her self-efficacy and thus her perceived self-control and thereby reduce her dyscognitions. Relaxation in hypnosis serves to counter-condition the physiological components of fear. Accordingly, different experiences should be made in hypnosis on the plane, which she can cope with positively—or which can even serve as counter-conditioning, such as eating something delicious. In connection with this, she should perceive her now realized self-control and her self-efficacy for coping with fear as contingent. Post-hypnotic tasks that include relaxation and self-efficacy should be set for support.

Therapy Implementation

Induction

Point fixation is carried out, the patient immediately responds to this with relaxation. As a *rest scene*, "sand beach" is chosen: beach, white sand, turquoise water, hammock and palm trees like in the Maldives. She reports very vivid and realistic imaginations during and after hypnosis. In the process, she increasingly experiences relaxation and as a result, she feels warm hands and feet.

Therapy Scene

In the following problem scene, she initially sits in the airplane by the aisle. After several relaxation rounds and corresponding positive suggestions, she feels comfortable there, a habituation occurs as she independently tries out different seats, walks around the aisle, etc. (= *self-efficacy*) and relaxes more and more. The unpleasant food smell she suddenly perceives in the scene causes her stomach discomfort. When she then switches back to the relaxation scene, she feels better, more relaxed in her stomach. After three repetitions, she finds the smell of food pleasant as spaghetti Bolognese, feels hungry, and eats with appetite (= *counter-conditioning*). Now she can order a cola on my suggestion and drink it with pleasure (= *self-control, counterconditioning*). In addition, she imagines a scene on my suggestion that enhances relaxation and her self-efficacy: flight preparations such as packing suitcases, checking in, takeoff and departure, and being relaxed with the *Everywhere Method*. The patient is surprised by the reality of her inner images and the positive changes in stomach feelings, smell, etc.

Therapeutic homework: She should apply the Everywhere Method in different situations, combined with the posthypnotic tasks for relaxation and self-control. For her safety, she asks for two more appointments.

Effects

For the real departure, she has slight travel fever, but feels relaxed during the flight. On the return flight, she was even more relaxed, without any negative thoughts.

Therapy repetition

Four years later, the patient asks for therapy appointments again, as she now has office trouble and is under stress in the now started studies and because of a bachelor's thesis. Added to this are family burdens due to deaths and severe falls. She is concerned that all of this could negatively affect her feelings on her flight to New York in two weeks, especially at takeoff. Thus, she is concerned that this flight could trigger the fear feelings she experienced back then, as her first flight experience with fear was also a long transatlantic flight.

Therefore, we repeat the treatment of the previous treatment then. In addition, there is a *cognitive restructuring*: she is asked, after prior agreement, to think of the albatross she knows from the Disney film, which makes her happy, so that the fear thoughts etc. immediately stop (= counterconditioning).

Posthypnotic task: She should apply the Everywhere Method whenever she already feels small signs of fear: as thoughts, nervousness, or stomach discomfort.

Follow-up

She was able to use the Everywhere Method and the relaxing imaginations of the beach on the outbound and return flight, enjoy the food on board, etc.—no problems occurred. It was agreed after the end of therapy that the patient will get back in touch if there is a need for treatment. Since she asked for a refreshment of the treatment for the second flight journey, it can be assumed that she continues to do well without fear.

Discussion

This patient reacts to a traumatic flight experience with conditioned anxiety of flying, followed by fears of losing control. The psychotherapy treatments with a colleague were likely aimed at cognitive restructuring according to the patient's descriptions and were certainly appropriate. Probably these interventions were not helpful because they left the patient more passive, offered no alternative actions, and ignored the physical reactions.

The sudden food smells occurring in hypnosis were not unusual. In hypnosis, hallucinations can arise relatively easily and spontaneously, the cause of which is not immediately apparent. In this case, it is probably the smells during the flight when food is being prepared and served. They then belonged to the holistic experience of the flight (VAKOG). This raises the question for the therapist of how to deal with it: negate or include? The decision is then made to include them as normal perception and, if possible, to use them therapeutically (= utilisation), in case she has an appetite for this dish, which was indeed the case. If the smell had been aversive, a suggestion would have been proposed that the smell is indifferent, i.e., negated.

Overall, it is again astonishing how quickly and directly short-term therapy works, even though strong fear conditioning is present here. The effective factors here consist of the multidimensional approach, in which the patient can try out under which stimulus conditions she feels comfortable on the plane (walking around, etc.), her olfactory hallucinations are physically included, and also the preparations for the flight are manageable for her and can be overcome without fear through the Everywhere Method. Overall, these are sequences of self-control and spontaneously experienced self-efficacy.

12.3.6 Case 13—Anxiety of Spiders Since Childhood

Exploration

At a congress seminar in Switzerland, a 71-year-old participant, a doctor, psychotherapist, and hypnosis expert, comes forward. We have known each other for several years through these hypnosis professional congresses.

Now, according to her own statements, she has found the courage to seek treatment for her strong fear of spiders. She has suffered from this since her childhood but kept it as secret as possible because she was embarrassed to have such fears. She lives in a house with a garden; spiders of different sizes are normal here. She is particularly afraid of the thick, large specimens with long hairy legs. When she sees these from a distance (approx. 3 m), she is then inhibited in her actions, e.g., passing by, shooing them away with a broom, etc. So she takes detours in the house to avoid having to pass them. Spiders are creepy to her, and she is disgusted by them; just thinking about them gives her goosebumps. She can observe and accept other animals, such as the (non-poisonous) snakes that occur in her garden, without fear.

Study questions

- Please create a behavioral analysis regarding the triggers and reinforcing conditions
- Derive a therapy plan from this.

Behavioral diagnosis/behavioral analysis

Here we have a classic fear conditioning, so that just the sight or the thought of spiders triggers strong fear reactions. The avoidance behavior results in a negative reinforcement of the fear and, in connection with the dyscognitions ("spiders are creepy etc."), maintains the fear problem.

Prognosis

Since the conditioned fear with strong avoidance behavior has existed for seven decades, the cognitive and motor behaviors have probably become very entrenched. Since the motivation for therapy is high—and also the belief in the positive effect of hypnosis, a favorable therapy prognosis can be assumed.

Therapy planning

Anxiety confrontation should take place to reduce anxiety, combined with counter-conditioning through relaxation. This confrontation takes place in sensu, i.e., in hypnosis. In connection with this, cognitive restructuring should be achieved by observing one's own change behavior, to assess spiders as harmless. Post-hypnotic tasks should contribute to the stabilization of behavior changes (freedom from fear).

Therapy implementation

Induction

As a hypnosis-trained professional, she responds very quickly to the induction.

Rest scene
She wishes her garden as a *rest scene*, but without spiders; she can realize this rest scene very well.

Therapy Scene
After just two confrontations, she can look at the idea of a spider from a relatively close distance with relative calm. She is very surprised at how her attitude towards spiders suddenly changed after the positive suggestion. After several repetitions and *independent adoption* of the intervention, she can even view spiders of different sizes calmly as typical inhabitants or even cohabitants of her house. Since she responds so well and quickly to fear reduction, she is now advised with the *posthypnotic task* to apply the *Everywhere Method* as needed, i.e., at the sight of a spider in the garden or in the house.

Study Question

- Is the treatment completed with this, or should further methods or suggestions follow?

Further posthypnotic suggestions should follow. So far, the suggestions have involved purely mental coping by looking at the spider. However, she should also be able to act concretely, e.g., when the spider approaches her or does not leave the house. So the posthypnotic suggestions also include concrete scenes in which she is active, e.g., chasing away the spider with a broom. She quickly accepts this suggestion and acts accordingly positively.

Follow-up
After a few weeks, she tells me over the phone about her ongoing successes: She can calmly and relaxedly walk past spiders or even put a water glass over them and carry them out. The lady is now 88 years old and still actively working. She is my dear hypnosis friend in Switzerland. Several times a year we exchange our hypnosis case experiences and she then also reports with great joy how indifferent she is to spiders. She can catch them with a glass and carry them out to the garden or bring them there on their spider thread. She can live with them "in peaceful coexistence," as she contentedly describes it.

Discussion
Here too, beyond the purely cognitive and passive solution (looking at the spider), concrete action models are worked on in hypnosis. With these motor success experiences made in hypnosis, the patient can act all the more easily in the real situation, because she only has to "retrieve" and process the motor engrams created in hypnosis in the real situation. Her now fear-free behavior is self-reinforcing.

The example (see also case 8) also shows that the age of a client for psychotherapy and hypnosis application does not have to be limited, as was perhaps assumed a few decades ago. The decisive factor is cognitive flexibility.

12.3.7 Case 14—Dental Anxiety Since Childhood

Medical History
A student, approximately 23 years old, has suffered from a great fear of the dentist since his childhood. It is primarily the fear of injections. The fear begins days before the doctor's appointment. As soon as he thinks about it, he becomes restless, notices stomach pressure and increasing nervousness. As soon as he sits in the treatment chair, he begins to tense up, sweat, etc. He knows of no other possible fears or burdens.

> **Study Questions**
> - Do the previous exploration information already provide clues to a diagnosis and possible treatment elements?
> - Create a behavioral analysis of the triggering and maintaining conditions of the problem.
> - With which interventions should one best start?

Diagnosis
Since the fear begins days before the dentist appointment, as soon as he thinks about it, the cognition "dentist" is probably the triggering stimulus for the subsequent chain of behavior, which at its end causes strong physiological reactions. The cognitions here are: anticipatory fears, dyscognitions about dental interventions, fear fantasies, etc.

Prognosis
Since there are no recognizable/remembered traumatic triggering events for the genesis of fear, the fears are primarily cognitively conditioned. The fearful thoughts are limited only to the expected dental treatment. The patient's range of behavior is not restricted by this. However, health care could be affected if he delays or neglects control and treatment appointments due to his fears. Since these are very limited fears in terms of pain expectation, a favorable therapy prognosis with short-term therapy is to be assumed.

Treatment Plan
An intervention to reduce anxiety primarily involves reducing anticipatory anxiety and dyscognitions. Therefore, the intervention should start at the beginning of the behavioral chain "thinking of…". The patient should experience these triggering thoughts in hypnosis (= stimulus confrontation) and learn to cope with them in

order to be "emotion-free" or even relaxed in the treatment chair. Ultimately, he experiences self-efficacy, which in turn reinforces the now new changed behavior. He should then apply this cognitive restructuring acquired in hypnosis in the real situation.

Treatment Implementation
He responds quickly to the *induction* with intense relaxation.

For his *rest scene*, he chooses a walk in the forest and experiences it vividly and intensely.

Therapy Steps
For the *stimulus confrontation*, we start with the idea that it is a few days before the appointment and he is thinking about the dentist visit. Discomfort now arises, which must be endured (= habituation and prevention of avoidance behavior). The switch to the rest scene is quick. In the next imagined scene (and the *suggestion* of positive change), he mentions, surprised, that his thoughts became more indifferent and he became calmer, until after about six rounds including self-control, he is completely relaxed. Even the following idea of sitting in the treatment chair waiting for the injection now triggers indifference. Accordingly, the *post-hypnotic task* is to practice the Everywhere Method daily and then apply it in the treatment chair.

Follow-up
Days later, the client reports as agreed that he successfully applied the method. He now feels fit for further dental treatments, has no more anticipatory anxiety, as he now has the Everywhere Method at hand to control his further possible feelings of fear and his excitement. Overall, the case dates back about 15 years.

Discussion
The case clearly shows that the cognitive trigger (thinking of..) is responsible for the development of anxiety. Even in the further potential fear confrontation "sitting in the treatment chair", anticipatory fears, i.e. cognitions, primarily have an effect. It may well be that this patient is predominantly cognitively controlled and therefore prefers cognitive problem solutions. However, it cannot be assumed that he uses a general or exclusive cognitive control. In the case of other fears, problems or experiences, he may apply other solutions appropriate for the situation or corresponding trigger.

12.3.8 Case 15—Anxiety of the Upcoming Operation

Medical History
A doctor who has been practicing for many years, about 55 years old, is afraid of his hip operation scheduled for a quarter of a year from now. Primarily, it is the fear of being at the mercy of others and losing control over himself and the actions

in the operating room that passes in the time between preoperative preparation and anesthesia. As a doctor, he knows how much unwanted things can happen, how much can be botched. He cannot report any other fears.

The patient clearly describes his concrete fear of a justified loss of control in the specific preoperative phase—the trigger is thus the cognition "loss of control". The patient's concrete medical experiences and fear-laden cognitions are the basis for the genesis of fear. His insider knowledge focuses him on the critical points in the course of preoperative preparation. Accordingly, he knows exactly until when he wants to maintain control in order to be able to intervene if necessary.

Study Questions

- Define the primary triggers and components of the described fear problem.
- What form of treatment do you suggest here?

Diagnosis

So it's not about dyscognitions, but about objectively justified control desires. The patient has clear ideas about his future behavior, to maintain control and remain capable of action until the end.

Prognosis

Since the patient can clearly formulate his goals and desired real behaviors and the operation is to be performed, there is no avoidance behavior. Thus, with the existing high treatment motivation, a favorable course of therapy can be expected.

Treatment Planning

The patient should be cognitively and emotionally enabled to continue to critically perceive his environment during the period in question from surgical preparation to the initiation of anesthesia, to ask critical questions if necessary, and to intervene. Accordingly, the therapy scene should be designed in which the patient retains control as long as possible. At the same time, he should be mentally and physically calm in order to be prepared for the subsequent operation. Posthypnotic tasks are intended to help maintain this relaxation and awareness of control before surgery in a quarter of a year.

Treatment Implementation

He reacts "normally" to the *induction* with relaxation.

He uses the common *rest scene* "beach" and responds very well with relaxation to the suggestions for it.

In the *therapy scene* in hypnosis, the patient is in the preparation room for surgery on the stretcher. He can withstand the tension and is—like many—pleased when the switch to the rest scene occurs. He finds it pleasant.

After the *suggestion* of *positive changes*, he is amazed at how calm he has become. It is particularly reassuring for him to experience that there is a satisfactory control method, as he has just learned. Thus, after a few repetitions, he receives the instruction to trigger the next rest scene himself by touching his wrist. That is, he soon gets the desired opportunity to *actively control the situation* and regulate his feelings himself. After a few repetitions, he feels sufficiently fit to bring about the rest scene with its relaxing effect himself and satisfactorily. Since the achieved effect of self-regulation for the operation is to be used only in a quarter of a year, it is necessary that the client regularly applies the Everwhere Method in the meantime, both in comparable situations associated with stress or excitement, but also for pure practice purposes. To stabilize this, *posthypnotic suggestions* are made to carry out this exercise every day or every other day in peace and with sufficient time—and before or during exciting or similar situations. Then later, of course with this practice success, he will successfully carry out this Everywhere Method also in the preparation room for the operation and be calm and composed.

Follow-up

One year after this treatment, the patient reports at the next hypnosis congress with great joy and also with a certain awe of the effect of the method about his interim approach and successes: He practiced the Everywhere Method relatively regularly and also successfully applied it in "critical" situations (e.g. when excited). This gave him the confidence to be able to maintain control over his feelings of fear and excitement. When he then came for preoperative preparation, he used the exercise effectively. Now the anesthetist asked for routine safety that it was probably his *right* hip that was to be operated on. The client vehemently disagreed, as it concerned his *left* hip. The situation he had feared had now occurred. The client immediately remembered my instruction or the *posthypnotic task,* to immediately initiate the relaxation using the Everywhere Method, which he immediately succeeded in doing due to his previous practice experiences. He immediately noticed that he had thus maintained the very necessary control over this critical situation. The correctness of his intervention was confirmed by the doctor (meekly) based on the X-ray image, which also confirmed him in his actions. To the anesthetist's surprise, he had clearly expressed his opinion about this sloppiness, but still remained calm. Thus, he also clearly told her that he was now also mentally ready for the operation and that premedication should be dispensed with. So, according to his wish, the anesthesia was immediately initiated. The operation was carried out without complications and the subsequent rehabilitation measures as well. Now, nine months later, this operation is forgotten for him and he can move without complaints. He had wanted to inform me about this a long time ago, but had misplaced my address. Overall, he is very happy about this intervention, which was so helpful for him.

Discussion

In this case too, the patient can provide very clear information about his fear and the required therapy goals. His fear is conditioned by his cognitions "I know what can go wrong." and remains predominantly limited to this area, does not generalize into other areas of life or control functions. Therefore, it may be easy to make relaxation and evaluation changes here. In addition, he wants to maintain cognitive control in the situation he defined. This narrowly and clearly defined behavioral goal makes it easier for him and the therapist to deal with posthypnotic tasks tailored to it.

The challenge was to maintain motivation to reliably apply the Everywhere Method and benefit from relaxation within the upcoming quarter until the surgery. His purely mentally experienced successes in hypnosis, the preoperative control to regulate himself, gave him the confidence to use it successfully in the real situation.

It is noteworthy that he was able to remain calm after the news of the hip mix-up, did not get angry or even decompensated. It may be that he has already mentally played through this scenario he feared several times successfully. But it could also be that the successful achievement of his goal was now reached, as he was able to clearly exercise control. From a learning theory perspective, it is assumed here that there is a relief and confirmation of his efforts over the past months, which caused a reinforcement of his entire approach and thus relaxation. The post-hypnotic order was now completely fulfilled to his satisfaction, he could then hand over his responsibility to other people like the surgeons.

12.3.9 Case 16—Anxiety After a Medical Mishap

Condition

Michael is 8 years old, attends the second grade of elementary school. He is afraid of injuries, pain, and medical sounds. Therefore, he strictly refuses doctor contacts.

Genesis

About four years ago, after a leg fracture, his plaster cast was finally to be opened. The doctor used a special motor saw very clumsily, causing him to injure Michael painfully and bleedingly on the leg, thus classically conditioning the aforementioned fears. Michael is very open and communicative, so it is possible to explore that he is primarily afraid of being "ambushed" by the doctor (as before) without warning. He therefore needs security and wants to maintain control over himself.

Study Questions

- Create a behavioral analysis of the development of fear
- and make therapy suggestions.

Diagnosis

As already shown, the fear of pain, injuries, and medical sounds is classically conditioned by the accident.

Due to these real conditioned fear experiences, there are anticipatory fears, which could not only concern possible pain, but fears of being ambushed by the treating doctor again unprepared, i.e., being helpless, losing self-control.

Prognosis

Despite the classical conditioning, there was no anxiety generalization. Also, so far no problematic experiences have been observed. This means that avoidance behavior and other reinforcements did not occur. These are signs that the fear and the associated cognitions etc. have not yet "solidified". Therefore, a good effect from short-term therapy can be expected. Michael can describe his problem remarkably accurately. There is also good and trusted communication with him. These are factors that suggest good cooperation and thus a favorable course of therapy.

Therapy Plan

The focus of treatment should be the recovery of self-control, combined with the reduction of anticipatory fear of losing this control and security. From the exploration, it is clear that Michael is very communicative and enjoys discussion. Therefore, an attempt should be made to bring about a cognitive restructuring in the sense of a reevaluation of the events and thus the recovery of self-control, such as through the Socratic dialogue. Thus, short-term hypnotherapy is suggested. Possibly, young Michael will be overwhelmed if he should only make purely cognitive changes. Accordingly, activities are sought that give him pleasure but are associated with noise, in order to experience noise without fear through self-control. Due to his age, it should be considered to also involve the parents as co-therapists (see below).

Therapy Implementation

In very committed conversations with me, he realizes that his event back then was a coincidence. Since he responds very well to arguments, the method of Socratic dialogue is attempted (see Sect. 6.1.4.2and 7.3.4). We work out that one cannot protect oneself from all coincidences—and there are also pleasant coincidences such as birthday surprises. After this cognitive restructuring, his fear of a sudden intervention has decreased. In addition, he is now suggested to verbally intervene in the feared situation himself and actively shape the situation. He should tell the doctor that he becomes nervous and anxious with sudden actions. Therefore, the doctor should explain to him step by step what he plans to do. The mere thought of this active participation gives Michael confidence. To further improve his central self-control, we practice visualization images for relaxation, which he can apply before the future doctor consultation (= posthypnotic tasks).

Effects

Through these therapeutic instructions, Michael quickly notices the effectiveness of his self-control activities.

Since Michael's fear (8 years old!) is also part of his family system, the parents must be used therapeutically supportive, especially so that Michael becomes aware that he is not left alone with his problem. In addition, the father can contribute therapeutically. (See also Sect. 6.2 and Case 10)

In the *parent consultations* in Michael's presence, his successful self-controls are additionally reinforced by the empathetic parents. He also has the certainty that he can always rely on the support of his parents, regardless of his own efforts.

It is now additionally recommended to reduce the fear of "medical noises" by having father and son do crafts together and use, for example, the drill. This way, Michael can control unpleasant noises himself and probably get used to them the fastest. A generalization of the effects on medical noises is to be assumed. Both agree to this. After a few sessions, Michael is free of fear and can endure the next medical intervention without anxiety.

Follow-up

In an agreed reporting period of about one year, the behavior remains stable. It had been agreed with the parents that they would report if there were any new problems—which was probably not necessary.

Discussion

Here too, a pain traumatization occurs, which generalized. In this child, cognitive restructuring and self-control strategies are so successful through conversation with him that further treatment methods are unnecessary.

12.3.10 Case 17—Panic Attacks in the Tram

Exploration

The patient is 23 years old, a student with her own apartment. In recent months, she has had such severe panic attacks on the tram that an ambulance had to be called. After she had calmed down again in the hospital within a short time, she could be discharged immediately.

She is suddenly and seemingly without reason attacked by the attacks and feels helplessly exposed to them. This leaves her no time to think about possible countermeasures.

The further exploration shows that she had a strong argument with her parents for the first time before the first attack. So far, everyone in the family had gotten along well and harmoniously. Only occasionally did minor differences of opinion arise; then both she and her parents tried to clarify or appease them as quickly as possible. In the triggering incident described above, however, both parties disagreed so much that no solution could be found and they parted in dispute. On the tram ride to her apartment, she was then overcome by the panic attack, followed by the blue light deployment of the ambulance.

Study Questions

- Create a behavioral analysis of the triggering and maintaining conditions of the problem.
- Through which behavior, which constellation, did the panic attack arise?

Diagnosis

It is clear that strong emotions in the form of guilt were triggered by the insoluble dispute with the parents. These then triggered an increased level of physiological arousal, which led to the reported panic attacks and emergency hospital admission. The first occurrence of the attacks took place on the tram, which led to a conditioning, so that now riding the tram, associated with the specific smells, general perceptions and memories of the emotions and cognitions at the time of the event, triggered the physiological fear reactions.

The trigger of her panic attack was the dispute with her parents, in which no common peaceful solution could be found. The family is described by the patient indirectly as harmony-seeking, loving and always striving for balance. Accordingly, she and her family never learned to deal with conflicts and to endure or later resolve existing differences or disharmonies. Therefore, only feelings of guilt, frustration, despair, fear of loss of love or depression could follow as resulting behaviors.

Prognosis

Panic attacks are often difficult to treat, as by definition causes are rarely or not at all found. Since the patient comes to therapy relatively quickly after the first attack, concrete triggers such as feelings of guilt could be assumed. This indicates a relatively favorable prognosis. On the other hand, several family members are involved in the problem. Here it seems problematic whether changes are possible solely through the treatment of this patient. Possibly, a longer therapy or even family therapy may be necessary.

Treatment Plan

Since the family conflict primarily involves the regulation of attributions and emotions, associated with dyscognitions, a cognitive method should be used here. The patient should relive the conflict scene with the parents in order to then work through different solutions. Accordingly, a confrontation with the parents and behavioral exercises for conflict resolution should take place in hypnosis.

Therefore, the patient should now receive a therapy scene, after which she should decide: a) for example, offer the parents a solution or b) apologize or c) give explanations for her behavior. To weigh these alternative possibilities, she now relives the confrontation in hypnosis and then decides to explain her concerns to the parents. (The other aforementioned therapy options should be mentioned later as appropriate.)

Therapy Implementation

Induction

The induction is followed hesitantly, even interrupted by her, as she cannot imagine being able to bridge the gap to her parents "through something like this". Therefore, it is explained to her that this is merely an initial procedure with which we will find and try out solutions more relaxed. She can then agree to this.

Rest Scene

The offered images like "*forest*" and "*sandy beach*" do not appeal to her. The rest scene "*mountain scene*" briefly described by me appeals to her, as she knows and has loved the mountains, the peace there and the snow on the mountains and slopes from a holiday stay. Accordingly, she reacts very relaxed to this. Probably she has now found trust in me and the announced method and can now cooperate more easily.

Study Question

- Based on what information should further procedures be planned and carried out?

Therapy Scene

According to the therapy planning, she experiences the three relevant behavioral alternatives in hypnosis and is then asked whether this is enough for her, because after all, she was clearly right in this dispute. Now she decides to apologize for her rough behavior, but still to stick to her opinion without feelings of guilt. And she asks her parents objectively to accept this. Accordingly, she presents this to her parents in this hypnosis scene calmly and determinedly.

Suggestionof positive change

She now experiences (without impulse from the therapist) how the parents struggle with her opinion, but ultimately accept it and everyone in the family is relatively happy about the discussion and its ultimately positive end.

Posthypnotic Task

The patient has now mentally worked out a solution with which she and her parents can be satisfied. This solution should now also be put into concrete action, as otherwise the difference of both opinions and thus the unresolved conflict as a trigger of fear would remain. Therefore, the posthypnotic task is to have the clarifying conversation with her parents at a time agreed with the patient.

Debriefing
The patient is very glad to have found the cause of her panic attacks and also opportunities for clarifying conversations with her parents. She also knows that this will be difficult, as her parents are very conservative and harmony-seeking. However, she now feels strong and capable of having these conversations.

Study Questions
- Has the therapy been successfully completed with this?
- What further steps might be necessary?

It would be beneficial if the patient could resolve her long-standing conflicts and disagreements with her parents. Family therapy sessions might be useful. Further appointments are offered to her for this purpose.

Follow-Up
The patient did not show up for her scheduled appointment after this session.

Discussion
The case shows how dramatically seemingly small differences of opinion can have an impact when there is no culture of argument, the sensitivity of the family system is high, or the tolerance for frustration is low. This often leads to pathological consequences.

It also becomes clear here that the combination of elements such as cognition, emotion, and attribution can trigger severe panic attacks, probably when the situation is assessed as hopeless or one experiences oneself as helpless.

The solutions suggested in hypnosis (apologize/explain/insist/etc.) are not unconditional fixed concepts. They only provide possible solutions derived from the patient's descriptions, which the patient should then select and test in a hypnosis scene. Often, one is blocked for solutions or thought impulses in such situations, or one has not yet been able to learn solutions in this area of conflict and now has to learn them under therapeutic guidance. Because at the beginning of therapy, a solution that is possible and acceptable for the patient must first be found. However, if these solutions are too simple or superficial, the therapist should point this out, then suggest more appropriate solutions and test them with the patient in hypnosis. A superficial solution would be, for example, if the patient gives in unconditionally out of guilt feelings or breaks off contacts with the conflict partner without discussion. The causes for further panic attacks or similar physiological behavior would then continue to exist.

According to the considerations for the prognosis, it was relatively unlikely that the patient could acquire so much social competence after one session to change long-standing and thus entrenched family structures and conflict potentials.

12.3.11 Case 18—Panic Attacks - Really Without Apparent Reason (?)

Condition

After a year of unsuccessful Psychotherapy with his patient suffering from panic attacks, the treating doctor asks me to take over the case soon, to apply my special method in anxiety therapy. Unfortunately, only a brief initial conversation is possible before the start of therapy.

Exploration

The patient is about 25 years old, a trained dental assistant, but she gave up her professional activity after a few years because she increasingly showed fears that she could not cope with, so she has been sick and therefore unable to work for about 2 years. She appears very shy and can tell me nothing about the nature, origin, and effects of her fears. Ultimately, the suspicion arises that she triggers her fears herself through negative thoughts.

Study Questions

- Would the short-term therapy possibly have been applied sensibly here?
- Are these informations sufficient to establish an appropriate diagnosis?

Beginning of Short-Term Therapy?

The patient's suffering due to her fears and her long-term unemployment may motivate the therapist's willingness to help, to finally apply an intervention to reduce anxiety. Treatment with hypnosis or even short-term therapy with suitable hypnosis suggestions can be tempting here. Since the therapist who has been treating her so far was unsuccessful with his method, this can be even more of an incentive to start anxiety treatment immediately. But hypnosis and suggestions are only permanently helpful if they are applied causally. This means after finding and establishing a diagnosis, i.e., after recognizing the effective causes.

Further Diagnostic Planning

The patient's previous information did not seem sufficient to derive a clear diagnosis, let alone an indication for a therapy method.

It should be clarified what her fears specifically consist of and what triggers her fears. To make use of the time until the next possible appointment in about 6–8 weeks, a personalized "questionnaire" is quickly designed for her on the PC. It contains questions about triggers, cognitions, emotions, coping strategies.

The following needs to be filled in:

- Time when the fear begins
- Fear content: why, what is the fear of?

- Scaling of fear intensity on a scale from 0 to 100.
- Fear scaling **before** and **after** this (possible) coping
- Can the fear be overcome? With what?
- Overall assessment of her situation

She is given numerous of these "forms" to fill out and send in each week. She agrees to this, slightly skeptical, but glad because something concrete is finally being done about her anxiety.

(Aside: In the case of such fears, which could even be described as panic, inirect or client centered therapy is quite contraindicated. Because the danger with this form of treatment is that one always circles around oneself with fears, which the patient did for over a year of treatment.)

As agreed, the patient sends me the completed protocols for evaluation on a weekly basis. During the waiting period until the start of therapy, it becomes clear:

- There is a great fear (about 80–90 scale points) **before** an action in general and decreases significantly by about 30–40 scale points **after** performing the action.
- The actions associated with fear are very simple in nature such as: cleaning the budgie's birdcage; buying groceries etc.

The conclusions and questions from this:

- These are very simple activities—why is the patient afraid of them?
- She always has anticipatory fears before an action.
- After the action, her arousal level immediately drops significantly.
- **Conclusion:** This is very unlikely to be panic attacks.

Exploration

When the treatment can finally begin, a conversation with the patient about these conclusions from her protocols takes place. In order to reduce her possible fear of failure, it is emphasized that her self-observations and protocoling are very helpful and can now shed light on the origin of the fear problem. She is very relieved about this. But why is she afraid of such relatively simple actions? Further exploration is carried out as to which actions cause her so much fear.

It slowly becomes clear: Her parents divorced when she was about 10 years old. Now the mother took over all household chores to spare her at least in this way. In agreement with the patient, a conversation with her mother now took place. She admitted very tensely that she had feelings of guilt towards her daughter because of the divorce and wanted to relieve and spoil her in everything.

Study Questions

- Create a behavioral analysis of the triggering and maintaining conditions of the problem.
- What therapeutic interventions do you suggest?

Diagnosis

It now becomes clear that the patient has *behavioral gaps* in many areas of everyday life. That is: She has acquired few action competencies and therefore always fears not being able to meet the demands of everyday life, to fail. For example, she couldn't even fry eggs or go shopping in the supermarket relaxed. Until now, the mother has reduced her feelings of guilt towards her daughter by supporting her daughter overprotectively. Thus, the feelings of guilt were negatively reinforced and remained, including spoiling the daughter. The diagnosis "panic attacks without a recognizable reason" is clearly refuted (see Fig. 6.6 or a similar constellation).

Prognosis

Anxiety treatment can only be successful if it addresses her significant behavioral gaps (= low everyday skills). This will only succeed with the help and cooperation of the mother. Therefore, it will depend on her whether the patient will gain the required independence. Depending on this, further steps such as vocational integration etc. will be possible.

Study Questions

- Which therapy methods are now sensible—for which person?
- When should short-term therapy be indicated for the treatment of anxiety?

Therapy Plan and Therapy Methods

The focus of the treatment is now clearly on methods to gain behavioral skills in order to reduce the existing behavioral deficits that have so far caused anxiety. In this context, *shaping* is useful, i.e., the gradual development of everyday skills.

Therapy Plan

The *daughter* must definitely learn everyday activities (e.g., shopping, cooking) in order to lose her fear of them = closing the behavioral gaps through skill acquisition and thereby increasing self-reinforcement. At the same time, the daughter loses comforts: she has less "free time" because she now has to help around the house. However, at the end of this relatively long procedure, she is ready to apply for a job without fear.

The *mother* would thereby lose the ability to spoil her daughter, in order to reduce her feelings of guilt. This could cause problems, because as the daughter becomes more independent, she would become "superfluous". That is, the feelings of guilt remain, the daughter's affection decreases = very strong losses for the mother, even loss of her purpose in life, possibly leading to depression. This can sometimes lead to the affected person (mother) wanting to prevent these losses and therefore reacting excessively with pampering—or breaking off the therapy to maintain the usual system.

Accordingly, the mother should now receive verbal affection from her daughter (and the therapist) when she guides her in closing her behavioral gaps. She can then be proud of how independent her daughter is becoming, in order to be fit for a job application without fear.

Therapy Implementation

Competence Training
The therapy therefore begins with training in everyday skills, e.g., in the household. In agreement with mother and daughter, a plan is drawn up according to which the mother instructs her daughter in these activities, which are gradually increased in demands over time (= habituation). Accordingly, as her daughter becomes more independent, the mother increasingly withdraws from her responsibility.

The *mother* is increasingly motivated in carrying out these exercise steps, because now she can develop a good conscience, as she is helping her daughter to become capable of living and free from fear.

The *daughter* shows—as was to be expected—initial resistance, as she now has to do more in the household and take on responsibility. Over time, however, she recognizes the great advantages of self-efficacy and autonomy; she achieves this after just a few weeks. Accordingly, she has completely eliminated the previously occurring anticipatory anxieties. She now even feels fit enough to apply again as a dental assistant. Now the conditions are created for the patient to be able to manage her everyday life without "panic attacks" and be fit for further measures.

Re-Integration—Therapy with the Hypnosis Short Method
After these successfully completed treatment steps, however, there are still "normal" fears of a job interview with a dentist. This is where short-term therapy comes into play: In hypnosis, she is relaxed and conducts a job interview. She experiences herself as confident, competent, and self-effective.

The *induction* and the *rest scene* are well implemented; in hypnosis, a behavior rehearsal takes place, i.e., a behavior training for the job interview.

This form of "hypnosis short therapy" works immediately; the patient is confident and self-assured. The patient now goes to the job interview relaxed and is immediately accepted. However, she ends her employment after 1-2 weeks because she finds the doctor not clean enough and sufficiently hygienic. The exploration of this reveals that the patient did not show any fears or avoidance behaviors in the dental practice, which would be possible after so many months of resumed work. Her decision to quit there was clearly objectively correct, well thought out, and clear. She could only be confirmed in this.

Fortunately, she had a new job offer after a few weeks, which she liked very much from the dentist and his team. She was highly motivated and was promoted after a few weeks due to her good ability to take over an independent work area!

Follow-up
There is no later discussion available; however, since the patient had great confidence in her abilities and her therapist due to her successfully concluded negotiation, she would certainly have contacted again if there had been any problems.

Discussion
Often the diagnosis of "panic attack" is made when immediate causes of the fears cannot be found. These can be so far back that they are no longer remembered, one has arranged oneself with the fear in the present, or the triggers are so subtle that they can only be found with a lot of patience and detailed work in the exploration.

The mother-daughter constellation is almost classic, because their disorders and social dependencies condition each other and thus maintain themselves in a loop. Therefore, an interruption had to be found here, which is usually associated with loss of reinforcement. These deficits must—as in the above case—be filled in order to achieve therapy successes. Then even a win-win situation arises for both people. The short therapy to reduce the relatively small fear of the job interview had an important, but only subordinate function here.

12.3.12 Case 19—Anxiety of Failure, Self-Doubt, Social Anxiety, Feelings of Inferiority

Preliminary remark
Case 19 (see below) forms the announced exception here, because the client's fear problems are primarily in the area of self-attribution and anticipated external attribution. The order of the therapy steps was also adapted to the client's sensitivities and the resulting methodological requirements. The comments in the text justify this then.

The exact reproduction of the therapy dialogue also shows that some steps may seem redundant due to their repetitions. Since the method implies clarifying and changing the relationship between the individual components of fear, this can only be done carefully and in small, repeating steps, which then always contain an improvement towards the therapy goal.

The verbatim transcript of my therapy session shows the results of the exploration (approx. 30 min) and then live the concrete communication during the entire therapy implementation (60 min).

The therapy part contains the complete text of client and therapist. The written text unfortunately cannot reproduce how calm and accepting, but goal-oriented the therapist speaks, but leaves the client her freedom for her answers.

For better understanding, the individual phases or steps of the method are marked in the text, so that readers can understand the procedure in detail. Additional comments are also inserted.

Exploration

Client (C): Mrs. W., 56 years old, academic with her own practice/office. Divorced; living in partnership.

She has professional fears of failure, "although I constantly further my education". She always has the feeling of not being enough, both privately and professionally.

She often thinks: "You could have done better. That's not enough yet." Is then very depressed about mistakes, thinks she makes more mistakes than others, which according to her evaluation "of course is not true." She thinks she is not lovable, does not meet the requirements of others.

Summary of the client's report

My mother was a housewife. When a child came, she gave up her studies and what she had not achieved, I should achieve.

I had a sheltered childhood, orderly circumstances. Until the start of school, I was extremely temperamental, full of zest for life. And then that was lost. Then there was only depression and sadness left. … Now I am already so old and want to get back the carefreeness. With the start of school, demands were made on me that I experienced as pressure.

Performance or top performance was always demanded of me. More than from others.

I always met the requirements, but then the bar was always raised—that was my impression. Mother's demands remained even after school, even during my studies.

Because of the sheltered environment, I had close contact with my mother and therefore a lot of communication with her. We often phoned. This way she could always exert pressure. When you have such a close relationship, you also want to be loved, praised, comply with it.

There was no rebellion; I tried to meet the demands.

I only noticed this when I was 30 with the first partner, because my mother was not satisfied with him, with his degree, his personality. She never did this directly, but more subtly. … When I spoke well of my partner, she was silent and didn't want to hear any more about it. Very subtle. I then separated from him.

My mother liked another partner. I then realized that we didn't fit together and separated from him. My mother took this very badly; she then disinherited me because of it.

That's when I noticed that this ran through my whole life and I felt oppressed. I could never satisfy her, I was rejected.

My mother then became seriously ill, I took care of her. When she died, she apologized to me. I accepted it, because I wanted her to have a good death.

My partner, with whom I have been together for ten years, is my support. He fully accepts me, supports me. He listens to everything.

Previous attempts at solution
She consulted group psychotherapy. I saw that every person carries their own burden. "That built me up. It was relieving to see. That helped me.

I then broke off contact with my mother for half a year. Then I felt extraordinarily well. I tried to talk to her. She then evaded, blamed it on the father."

T What would you most like to say to your mother today? Or what would you most like to do differently today? If you had had a magic wish back then. What would you have wished for then?

K I would have wished that they hadn't put pressure on me at school. She should have said: "Have fun, you don't always have to get A's, have friends. Choose a profession that you enjoy, that your heart is attached to. Live in your life, don't just perform."

T My suggestion: Shall we take a look at what you would have most liked to say to your mother?

K Yes.

Considerations for Diagnosis
Due to the excessive performance demands of her mother, the patient internalized her evaluation system, developing social anxieties, fear of failure, and feelings of inferiority in order to meet her own and external demands, professionally or privately. She never learned to assert herself against these demands and to develop her own positive self-evaluation. This results in her fears of failure and fear of failure with tendencies towards despair and depression. It gives the impression that she can hardly perceive herself as a person or physically (Fig. 12.1).

Prognosis
The problems have existed for a very long time and are associated with numerous expectation patterns, evaluations, etc. in the family system. Therefore, short-term therapy will probably only enable new perspectives on correlations or evaluations. This can then be the beginning of a longer treatment.

Therapy Planning—Therapy Goals
The client should recognize the emotional, cognitive, and physical effects of her negative self-evaluations and social fears of negative external evaluations. Her attempts at solutions were so far too weak and very rare to bring about a positive self-evaluation. Therefore, she should have the opportunity to experience in hypnosis how she achieves and feels liberating solutions. Accordingly, she should

Self-assessment -	assumed External assessment	- Emotion -	Motivation -	Imagination -	Physiology
I cannot suffice.	She feels inadequate	Fear of failure Despair Depression	I want to do even better.	?	? see Therapy

Fig. 12.1 Sequence of individual phases of fear.
Fear consists only of attributions, emotions, and motivation; imaginations and physiological reactions do not seem to be perceived

recognize that she should re-evaluate her performance and performance expectations of herself. For this, she should recognize that she can meet and accept her demands—also in comparison with other people—and experience herself as valuable.

Since she has so far only lived according to the evaluations and expectations of her mother and according to the evaluations of other people she assumed, she should recognize her own values in hypnosis, possibly in dialogue with her mother, and live freely according to them.

Preparation—Explanations

T I will now explain to you how I will proceed later, how we will work together later. I will ask you shortly which scene is relaxing for you. And then a scene that was oppressive for you back then. Then I will tap you on the shoulder at this scene. Is that okay? (When K agrees, he briefly touches her shoulder). In the other case, when you relax later, then I will just press here a bit (touches her wrist). Agreed? (K nods.).

Exploration for the Rest Scene

For Mrs. W., the Baltic Sea beach is pleasant, as she has been there several times: shallow shore, sandy beach, pleasantly warm sun. In addition, it is explored whether she can walk with her feet in the water. This is to find out whether there is possibly fear of the water, fear of loss of balance, or cold feet—but this is not the case here. Already during this exploration (with VAKOG, see Sect. 2.5.8) it becomes clear from the client's facial reactions that she can vividly imagine these scenes.

Therapy Implementation

- **Step 1: Induction**

The finger fixation method is used; the client responds to it immediately and is in deep relaxation after three minutes. This step takes 3 minutes.

- **Step 2: The Rest Scene—Relaxation**

The client experiences deep relaxation on the Baltic Sea beach; she likes sitting in the warm sand the most, which is then particularly emphasized. This step takes 4:12 min.

- **Step 3: Learning the body signals for relaxation**

The client cannot name a specific body part for relaxation, but feels very comfortable and relaxed overall.

- **Step 4: Learning the Everywhere Method**

The client has reported a lot in the exploration so far. To relieve her, the Everywhere Method is therefore only introduced in step 13, when she should apply it directly.

- **Step 5: The therapy scene—its triggers—learning to differentiate**

T (Puts finger on the shoulder.) You are now sitting opposite your mother and can finally tell her what you have always wanted to say. You see her vividly in front of you. Her typical hairstyle and clothing. …
K I feel a bit sick when I imagine that.
T Where do you feel it the most?
K In the stomach.
T Yes. Put your hand on it. … Please describe it in more detail.
K I want to tell her something, but before I say it, I just feel sick.
T Can you please endure it a bit. … What would you like to do now? … Run away?

- **Step 6: Perception of the *body signals* for relaxation**

(Implementing this step immediately after step 5 would have interrupted the aversive physical condition experienced in step 5. This would have promoted symptom-promoting avoidance behavior. Therefore, this step only takes place after step 8.)

- **Step 7: Enduring the aversive situation**

K Yes.
T You try to endure it now. … How are you doing with it. I am with you and you try to endure the feeling in the stomach for a while. And how is it?
K It's okay. (Overall about 60 s)

- **Step 8: Learning to switch quickly between both scenes**

T Yes, great. Now we switch again. I take the hand away (above) and you switch to the beach (wrist touch). … It is important that you can switch quickly. You are now back on the beach on the Baltic Sea. It is beautiful, sunny weather, you hear the waves and feel completely comfortable. … And now look at your body. Where do you notice something that is good for you and makes you feel comfortable? … It can be the forehead, the face, the neck, the chest, the stomach, the legs. Depending on how you notice it. ….

K Warmth.

- **Step 6: Perception of the *body signals* for relaxation**

(An attempt is now made again to locate the body signals for relaxation.)

T Where do you notice them? …

K Overall.

T Overall. Hm. … Can you place your hand somewhere where you say: "There I feel it particularly well, the warmth"? That does me good. …. Overall?

K Hm.

(Note: The client cannot specify a particular location of her positive feeling. This is rare, but it will not affect the further course.)

- **Step 8: Learning to quickly switch between both scenes**
- **Step 9: Suggestion of the perceived positive change**

T Then please try to hold on to this beautiful feeling of warmth: "This is my beautiful feeling. That does me good." We will also use this later. … O.k.? This is my beautiful feeling. I feel comfortable there. Please hold on to this for a while. … Great. … Now we switch back to the other scene. And please put your hand on the spot that was important earlier. And now notice what has already changed positively in the meantime.

K Well, at the moment I don't feel sick.

T Great! … So—how is it now?

K Calm.

T Loose in the stomach?

K Hm.

T Good. … And … You are sitting or standing opposite your mother. What can you tell her now? What can you do or say now that you have wanted to do for a long time?

K (20 sec) Why have you always pushed me?

T That sounds quite fearful? … But you can say it after all! Right?

K Hm.

T Is that already progress? I think so.

K Hm.

- **Step 10: Perception of the positive change and self-efficacy**

T Yes, good. Notice: You have now dared to say what you might not have been able to before. … And how does that feel in your stomach now?

K Good.

T Good, right? Great! … (Takes finger off the shoulder.) And now we switch back to the relaxation scene (now grabs the wrist)…. and notice: the whole body is well-being. You feel comfortable, relaxed and enjoy it. … It's wonderful to switch off like this. To sit or stand by the sea. To feel the warmth and relax wonderfully. You feel the warmth all over your body … Yes?

K Hm.

T Good. Hold on to that for a few seconds so that your body also remembers it. That you are completely relaxed. … (Touches the shoulder) Now we switch back to the other scene. And now look at what has changed even more positively. … Feel again on your stomach and also in your thoughts. … What has continued to change positively?

K I would say: "I want to get out of here. I want to get away from you."

T Tell her that: Your mother is sitting across from you and you tell her.

K (Somewhat hesitant.) "I don't want any more interference."

T Yes. … How do you feel when you say that?

K Good!

- **Step 11: Perception of self-efficacy and body signals**

T Yes. Where do you feel that most clearly?

K The body is light, lighter.

T Yes. Great! Enjoy the feeling, because you realize, you have now expressed it. I may have given prompts, but you have now expressed it. … You dared to say it. Yes? … Please hold on to that feeling. … Then we switch (finger from the shoulder; touch on the wrist.). You notice: You are back in relaxation, feel the warmth again on your body and enjoy being in the sun, feeling the warmth … hearing the sea … maybe tasting the salty air … all over your body… Are you feeling good with it?

K Hm.

T You're enjoying it like that. Great.

K (Nods.)

- **Step 12: Repetition loops, starting with step 7**

T (Shoulder touch) Then I switch back to the other scene. … You are again facing your mother. What has now further positively changed? … Look further. … See how you behave and how you feel about it.

K Distance.

T Yes, distance. … And does the distance do you good?

K (spontaneously) Yes.

T Great. … Where do you feel that?

K I feel lighter.

T Lighter. Great. … And what do you want to do now? Do you want to say something or do anything?

K Leave.

T Leave. Yes. … Just turn around or say something?
K No. Don't say anything.
T And what does it do to you when you now say: "O.k., I just want to leave."? What kind of feeling do you have with it?
K … Freer. …
T Free. Super. … Do you also notice that physically somewhere? Look and see if you notice that physically somewhere. The feeling of freedom, looseness. … Is that feeling okay?
K (nods.)
T Good, great. Then hold on to that again. You achieved that yourself. By behaving the way you just did, you caused this feeling of freedom in yourself. … Then we can switch back to relaxation (touching the wrist.) You can get some distance again by feeling completely relaxed, comfortable and wonderfully able to switch off. … Feel the warmth in your face, on your shoulders, on your chest … when the waves come and go … maybe sit in the sand and feel the warmth while sitting and enjoy just looking into the day. … Yes? … Is that pleasant?
K (Nods.)
T Yes. Great. It's very important that you feel completely comfortable and enjoy it a lot. … So, now I'm switching back to the other scene (finger on the shoulder.) And what do you notice, what has changed even more positively? …
K My mother is not there anymore.
T Yes. Where did she go? … Did she leave or just vanish into thin air?
K She's gone.
T Became uninteresting?
K Probably. (hesitant).
T Yes? But you don't quite trust it? … But it's a bit of a relief for you to notice, you don't see her anymore.
K Hm.
T Yes? Is it maybe like this—I don't want to suggest anything to you—"I managed to make the image disappear—I can control it myself, that the image is not there, which otherwise bothered me?"
K (Nods.)

- **Step 11: Reinforcement of self-efficacy**

T Yes, super. That's already another success. That you can control the image yourself … and thus control your well-being yourself. … Hold on to that: "This is my success. I achieved that. No one can take that away from me. This is my achievement, which I personally make. … I was able to assert myself. I was able to behave the way I want and can distance myself from the image of my mother. … Is that so?
K (Nods.)
T And what does that do to you. Where do you feel that?
K Unusual.

T Unusual … In which direction: unusually pleasant or unusually strange or threatening?
K Relieving.
T Is that something new, something nice?
K (Nods.)
T Yes, excellent. Hold on to that. This is something that **you** have achieved. With your ideas. With **your** thoughts. Please hold on to that very clearly for yourself. … Yes, hold on to it very clearly. (Touches wrist). This is **your** success. It's as beautiful as the relaxation scene. Yes … "*I am increasingly comfortable with the fact that I can do good for myself.*" Yes?
K Yes.

- **Step 9: Suggestion of the perceived positive change**
- **Step 10: Perception of the positive change and self-efficacy**

T My suggestion: Let's look at the scene again (touches shoulder). … What else has changed positively?
K I'm floating.
T Like on cloud nine?
K Not that extreme.
T But relieved—something like that?
K Hm.
T If you often heard in the past "I can't be enough" or ask yourself the question: "Is it enough?" What could you tell yourself now instead? … With this positive feeling that you just experienced: "I can control my own feelings and detach myself from the negative." … What sentence could you then tell yourself?
K (10 sec.) I don't know.
T It's a difficult question indeed. A suggestion I could make: Could you perhaps say: "With everything I have done or can do, that's okay. … That's enough. That's okay, that's even good." … See if you could think or say that about yourself.
K Difficult.
T Is this something completely new for you?
K Hm.
T What would be particularly difficult about it?
K … I think it can always be better.

- **Step 11: Reinforcement of self-efficacy**

T … That might be possible. Anyone can say that about themselves. … Let's switch back to relaxation (touches wrist). … That you are again by the sea and feel completely comfortable and balanced. … In doing so, gain a little distance from your doubts … and are on the beach and relaxed—and enjoy it. … And now let's just look at the scene again (touches shoulder). … And my suggestion is that you take a brief look back at the past and see what you have achieved. … You completed your high school—you completed your studies—and as I can guess, you did it quite well … You have your professional training, are practicing, have your clients and you are doing great in your profession. … Can you say that?

K 90%.

T Good. But 90% is good! … But that's not good enough for you? … Where do you feel that in your stomach right now? How does it feel at the moment?

- **Step 7: Enduring the aversive situation and attempting a cognitive restructuring of self-assessment**

K Feeling a bit sick.

T … What is causing you stress now?

K … That I don't want to lie.

T Yes, good. You're not supposed to. Otherwise, you would be lying to yourself. Heaven forbid; no one wants that. … I am now entering into negotiations with you. Earlier you said, 90% is fine. What would happen if you said: "I'll try 95% fine."? What would happen then? … Would that already be lying? Or would it be more like trying out—and I can live with that?

K … Hm. … Everyone is allowed to make mistakes, I think from time to time.

T Yes, okay. That's right, otherwise we would all be superhumans. … And you can also allow yourself to make mistakes from time to time. Yes? Good!

K … Hm.

T And could you accept that about yourself?

K Hm.

T Yes, good. And at what percentage would we be then? …. How would you feel at 95%?

K … I don't know.

T Would it be a struggle to allow that? Yes? … My suggestion: Also endure a bit whether you could be better than 90%. Whether that would be imposture for you. Or could you accept it like that?

K Difficult. …

- **Step 9: Suggestion of perceived positive changes**

T O.k. … Let's just switch back to relaxation (touching the wrist). It's not supposed to become stress for you. … Switch back. Notice your relaxation … at the Baltic Sea, where you feel comfortable, where you are doing well. … And now let's switch again (touching the shoulder) and see what has further changed positively. … Or whether you can say "90%! That's a lot. I trust myself that much. Man, great. 90% is also a lot. I can be quite satisfied with that".

K Yes!

T Would that be a success? … Compared to before—how would you have assessed it then?

K It's okay.

T So you can say: "Everyone makes mistakes. Me too. But I trust myself. 90% is a good rate. I can stand up well for myself. Good. Great. I agree with that. I can be satisfied with that."

K Hm!

- **Step 11: Reinforcement of self-efficacy**

T … What does it do to you when you perceive it like this? Think for yourself? Or possibly even be able to express it?

K Such a light feeling of happiness.

T Great! And please hold on to that.… "I notice, 90% of my activities are fine. I'm satisfied with that… Not just satisfied, but I can also be happy with that for myself. 90% is actually a lot!" … Yes, … not resigning, but … I think anyone would be envious and satisfied if they could say, 90% of their activities are fine. Right?

K (Nods.) …

- **Step 13: Self-control, Self-regulation**
- **Step 4: Learning the Everywhere Method**

(Now—as explained after step 6—the *Everywhere Method* can be applied in the overall context.)

T Try to accept that for yourself as well. … Maybe even that you can formulate it as a sentence for yourself. … (Removes finger from shoulder).

Now we're doing something new: Touch your own wrist. Just like I did. And now switch to your beautiful relaxation scene on your own. … You are at the sea, feeling good … it's about the same as before, only now you're doing it yourself, triggering the relaxation yourself with your hand. You will be able to do this yourself in the future, if you want it again … Whenever you want to be relaxed, you can practically switch on your relaxation in this way. … That means, you can touch your wrist like this anywhere, if you want to feel safe. That's why I called the method "Everywhere Method"; it works everywhere, so you can relax. … And when you are relaxed enough and feel good, let go of your wrist again. That's my signal that it's my turn again.

K (approx. 20 sec.)

T Now I give the signal to switch again (touching shoulder). So you know again what you can say, what you could think. … "I can be satisfied and happy for myself, 90% of my activity is fine. … This might be something new for me, that I can see so much positive for myself. But I notice it: that's me, who can see it like that. … Believe that for yourself … that you have such a picture: 90%. A lot, a lot of my things, they are good and others find them good too." … How do you feel about that?

K Unusual.
T Unusual—but as I understand it, pleasant. … Enjoy the feeling: It's unusually pleasant." … Also a bit liberating?
K Yes (nods).
T Very important! … Look for the feeling on your body.
K On the stomach.

- **Step 11: Reinforcement of self-efficacy and body signals**

T Good. Suggestion: Also put your hand on it, on that spot. … So you notice: Even my stomach has got it. I can see myself positively, can evaluate myself positively. I am worth a lot to myself! … I can distance myself from the past. I am worth a lot to myself. Not because others say so, but I have my self-worth for myself. … Right?
K (Nods vigorously,)
T A new feeling, a beautiful feeling. Hold on to it. "That's me. I can think and feel that." …
K Yes.

- **Step 14: Self-control of coping strategy**
- **Step 15: Stabilization of self-efficacy**

T Then please switch back, reach for your wrist, switch back to the other scene, so you can relax again, because even beautiful things can sometimes be a bit exhausting. Therefore, switch to the relaxation situation.
K (Grabs her wrist).
T Please hold this for about 20 to 30 seconds, so you notice that you are relaxed again. … It's important that you can switch back and forth. …
K (Raises hand = scene is over.)
T Now put your hand back on your stomach, so you can produce your own beautiful feeling. Now you can say: "Yes. I can produce my own pleasant feeling. I trust myself. I am enough for myself. What I do is okay for me. This feeling is new to me and beautiful and relieving." … Right?
K (Nods.)
T … and do you notice that something continues to change positively? That something is always getting a little better?
K (Nods).
T And what do you notice now that has changed positively?
K … Pleasant.
T Pleasant. Yes. … Can you also take this into your everyday life?
K I hope.
T Since this is new for you, you should somehow include it in your daily routine, so that you can bring up this beautiful feeling for yourself more often during the day. So that you notice that the new, beautiful thing belongs to you.

… Where could you integrate this about 1-2 times or more into your daily routine?

K Before falling asleep …

- **Step 16: Posthypnotic Task**

T Great. … Then please imagine a situation: You are in the bathroom, getting ready for bed. Do you have a specific bedtime ritual?

K I read gardening books.

T Great. So you can switch off nicely. … How about if you either before, during or after the gardening book tell yourself: "Great, I'm doing well. To this extent, I have made a new experience with myself. I can think positively of myself. Isn't that nice!" … When would be the best time? Before you start with the gardening book or in between, when you tell yourself: "Now I imagine again what new experience I have." Or, after you have read, you close the book and tell yourself: "Now I think again about my beautiful experience. And then I turn to my side and snuggle in."

K Yes, like that.

T Then please imagine it exactly like that. That in the evening, when you go to bed, you come out of the bathroom, lie down in bed, take your gardening book or your books … and look up certain things about certain plants or flowers or treatments of plants. That in itself is already a nice relaxing thing. … Imagine it vividly.

K (Nods.)

T And then you tell yourself: "Now I have read enough about it. Now I put my book or the magazine aside and now I imagine my new experience again. … I can see myself positively. This is something completely new. And I enjoy it now. I realize, I can accept what I do. That's great. I can rate this as good for myself … and accept myself, just as I am. This is a beautiful, new feeling. With this, I can snuggle up and sleep well." … Yes?

K Yes.

T Then please switch back to the relaxation situation, touch your wrist again … feel your relaxation … you already know this. … We are slowly coming to the end. … I would now like you to switch again and think about your evening scene: that you go to bed … fluff up your pillow, take your garden book and read interesting things, feel good and … when you have read enough and are tired, snuggle up and say: "Great, I have had a new positive experience with myself. I have seen in myself that the majority of my things are good and right. I can accept this for myself … and this is beautiful, this new feeling of life." … Please imagine this very vividly again … okay?

K Hm.

T And then you turn around with this beautiful feeling onto your sleeping side. Turn off the light … and sleep.

K (Nods.)

- **Step 17 Termination of Hypnosis—Positive Ending**

T I will count backwards from three to zero and you will then feel relaxed and comfortably active. … Three; you clearly hear my voice as now. Two: You are here in this room, on this chair. One: *You will feel relaxed and active when I say it, and feel confident about what you will think and feel about yourself soon.* And zero: You open your eyes. (= Posthypnotic suggestion).

K (Opens eyes.)

T Now I will be quiet for a while so you can arrive here.

K (After about 1 min.) Was good. …I've never had anything like this before. As if one has looked inside. But I still felt that I was here. Was not completely gone. As if one looks inside with the eyes, does not look outside. That's what it felt like. …

- **Step 18: Debriefing**

T Pleasant? (The therapist wants to focus the perception on positive content.)

K I felt a bit sick. I had some fears. I thought: "Oh", initially had the feeling: "Can this work at all?" As I got scared again and felt sick again. But then it got better over time.

T You also noticed: "I didn't let go!". … At the beginning, many have this fear. But if you endure it for a certain time—I was with you all the time—then you notice: the fear decreases.

K Exactly. At first, I had the feeling that it wouldn't work at all. There was always the fear. But then it gradually got better.

T You know, the therapist has to be patient. But he knows how it works.

K Hm.

T You noticed that; I was friendly-unyielding. Enduring does something.

K Hm.

T You noticed that as well.

K Yes!

T If you had said it hurts and I had then stopped, we would have already lost.

K Hm.

T You did the opposite of usual: endure. … What else did you notice?

K I was amazed that you still feel the environment. I thought, when you see it on TV, that you are like under general anesthesia. But that's not true. You still have a sense of the environment and still have one foot somewhere else. But you are not completely somewhere else. … At first, a third of the time, the fear always wanted to be against it. … That it takes quite a bit to get there somehow. But in the end, it was good.

T Can you name the fear?

K I don't know, I can't. No. It was against it. Against what was happening. It didn't want to get involved, the fear. Something like that.

T Let me put it this way: Leaving the usual pattern also hurts?

K Yes, maybe.

T Even if it was uncomfortable. You must have read about it; about the canary that was always in the cage and then the door was open and it got scared. Because it's something new, something unfamiliar.

K Maybe that's why. Exactly!

T You noticed, I didn't let go. How did you feel about that?

K Sometimes I couldn't describe it properly. I could imagine the room. But what kind of feeling I had there. … To fully engage in the situation is not that easy. You notice that you are in it, but then in the moment when you describe it or have to say something, you are even more in it. That's not that easy. I had a bit of trouble with that.

T Trouble remembering or because it then becomes uneasy?

K As if I always shy away from going into the situation one hundred percent. As if I try to evade a bit.

T Because it could hurt as much as before?

K I don't know. …

T You noticed, I didn't let go. How was that for you?

(The therapist insists here to explain the principle of avoidance behavior or the effect of enduring as counter-conditioning or habituation so that the client can understand and internalize the effect of enduring.)

K It was okay. Otherwise, I would have completely withdrawn from the event. So I was forced to continue. That was good. Especially in the end, it was good. I really noticed how I was feeling better. So there was a positive feeling. Therefore, it was good not to let go.

T You know, sometimes I experience that some people get annoyed when I don't let go. But I know what matters. As a therapist, you don't always make yourself popular when you don't always stop at the points where the other person says "ouch". … But I would feel the same way the other way around.

K Good.

- **Step 19: Therapeutic Homework**

T Now to the homework I would like to give you. Try to do this Everywhere Method a couple of times a day.

K A couple of times?

T Yes, just to refresh your relaxation. You noticed, it's quite simple. Just press the hand. … You can apply this in almost any situation. … This way you stay in training. My request would be that you do this at least once a day, at the latest when falling asleep, as we discussed earlier. That you ritualize believing in yourself.

K Hm. I had to overcome myself. …

T Did you feel under pressure in any way?

K At first, yes. Afterwards, I felt good. … I think if I stick with it, it will definitely be good.

T I believe so too. … My suggestion is that you can continue to contact me by phone if you have any questions.
K I will write down the sentences. Otherwise, I will forget them.
T Very good idea!
K There are only four sentences.
T You can almost use them like life formulas. They help tremendously. … Can we finish at this point?
K Yes.
K These are the sentences: "I am worth it.—90% are right—This is okay for me." I will put this on my bedside table.

(Note: One can hardly wish for a better positive conclusion of the therapy session, which even includes self-instructions.)

Follow-up

For this case, there is only a follow-up period of 6 months. The client continues to strive to perceive herself positively.

> After the very detailed case demonstration, the approach and conversation methodology of the therapist in the individual therapy phases became clear. Therefore, the following case examples should again be presented in a condensed form.

12.3.13 Case 20—Exam Anxiety—Fear of Assaults

Medical History

The psychology student, about 22 years old, is in a female psychotherapeutic treatment with a colleague due to trauma from a rape a few years ago. Since this assault, she has been afraid in many situations, especially of men, and no longer trusts them. She is a few weeks away from her intermediate exam, is afraid of it and asks for psychological support for this as well during her trauma treatment. For the therapy of exam anxiety, the female colleague asks me to take over this part of the treatment, as I have extensive experience with it, including the suitable intensive short-term therapy. The patient initially hesitates, as she now has to temporarily accept therapy from a man. After being informed by the colleague about my specialty "therapy of exam anxieties" and thus an acceleration of her treatment in this area is to be expected, she agrees. With the colleague, I clarify that abrupt movements and too close physical proximity of a male therapist could unsettle her.

> **Research Question**
>
> - How should the male therapist behave in such a preloaded situation?

Diagnosis
This is a case of frequently occurring exam anxiety, which is not generalized and only situation-dependent.

Prognosis
Based on the existing diagnosis, the treatment prospects are favorable (also based on the therapist's treatment experiences). The presence of the male therapist, a physiologically increased arousal level, can complicate treatment in addition to the existing tensions of examination and traumatization.

Treatment Planning
It is considered that it would be sensible to keep the seating distance to her as large as possible. Additionally, it is important to me not to touch her shoulder and wrist; they could cause fear, or at least mistrust, in a client with this background problem—both counterproductive for the planned treatment.

It is also planned to inform the patient of all details of the treatment beforehand and to explain their effects precisely. That is, she will not only always be informed, but she will be explicitly asked to intervene or ask questions immediately if something could unsettle her. This includes the explanation of the individual steps and the basic information about hypnosis and the patient's forms of experience. As a psychology student, she will be very critical, especially of hypnosis.

With expectation anxieties, the temporal distance to the relevant event (examination) is essential; as the event approaches, fear usually increases. Accordingly, the patient should learn the *Everywhere Method*, which she should already apply when small signs of anxiety such as restlessness occur.

Treatment Implementation
In the first session, she is relatively brusque and monosyllabic towards me, appears somewhat hostile. She mentions how many, many pages she has to read for the exam, much more than was customary (with me) years ago. This was a more or less direct attack on the therapist and his former study competencies. (Such aggressions towards therapists are part of the patients' defensive behavior (see Sect. 4.4.1.1). Also, in the sense of the overall therapy goals, the therapist should be experienced by her as a positive and non-aggressive male person.) This attack is simply ignored.

Since any kind of approach was to be considered potentially threatening for the patient, a modification was made: Instead of my finger pressure on her shoulder, she should touch herself on the shoulder; also, the switching by grasping the wrist should be done by herself. She cooperated well in this way.

Due to her extreme negative experiences with a man, the patient needed my continuous and reliable, indeed predictable, action. How could she now close her eyes for hypnosis and trust me during this time that I as a man would not become intrusive in any form, could come too close? On the one hand, like all other patients with mistrust or fear of hypnosis, loss of control, etc., I gave her the option to keep her eyes open or close them whenever she decides. This *freedom of decision* alone allows almost all patients to close their eyes after a while. Furthermore, my plan was not to move or make any noise during her eye closure, such as causing clothing rustling through arm movements—and thus causing fear or unease in this patient. This was the strenuous part for the therapist, having to sit without the slightest movement during the approximately 30-minute intervention. But in this way, the patient could experience after opening her eyes that the therapist was sitting just as he was before her eye closure and was therefore reliable.

History of Exam Anxiety

The *anamnesis* revealed that she was able to prepare well for the exam and only needed relatively few learning tips. The focus was therefore on my special short therapy, to reduce her anticipatory anxiety about the exam situation.

Research Question

- State your behavioral analysis and the therapy methods derived from it.

Diagnosis and Treatment Planning

Since learning and preparing for the exam is well realized, this is a case of simple expectation anxieties that occur when thinking about the exam or parts of it and bring slight discomfort. Self-evaluations and motivation are not affected. Accordingly, she should practice relaxation with the Everywhere Method and the quick switching from negative thoughts to relaxation. The exercise of actively induced self-control by her is in the foreground.

Therapy Implementation

Induction

She responds relatively quickly to the induction, can close her eyes and relax.

Rest Scene

The rest scene "Forest Walk" is desired. Since a forest could be anxiety-inducing for a patient with a history of assault, a detailed exploration was carried out as to what this forest must look like, etc., to be relaxing. The suggestions tailored to this cause her to experience good relaxation.

Study Question

- Plan the further steps of the therapy.

Therapy Scene

Since the patient primarily has anticipatory anxieties until the start of the exam, a scene is selected according to her descriptions in which she is a long time, then a short time before the exam and can remain calm through the *Everywhere Method*: she clearly notices that she can practice self-control in the situation and is not at its mercy.

With her strong basic problem, she is given a lot of time for the exercise, which is also repeated more often.

Effect

The entire treatment of exam anxiety took about 5 sessions, during which she gradually gained confidence in her self-control abilities, which she had completely lost during her rape.

Follow-up

The patient passed her intermediate exam with calmness and good grades. As the referring female colleague then reported, the most important experiences for the patient were probably that a man behaved reliably, predictably, she could increasingly trust him and he was even supportive and therapeutically helpful for her. At the same time, her experience of exercising self-control again in a stressful situation was very important to her. This significantly accelerated her overall treatment of PTSD.

Discussion

With the existing serious history and basic problem, the planning and implementation of short-term therapy was less in the foreground than the planning of the methodical approach in the overall situation "presence of a man"—"building trust"—"giving up or allowing control" and "regaining self-control.

This shows how complex a supposed short-term therapy sometimes has to be designed.

12.3.14 Case 21 Aggressions due to Lack of Self-Control

Preliminary Remark

This case has already been reported earlier (Kossak 1993, 2001); it is to be presented below with other focuses and within the concept conveyed here.

History

The principal of a secondary school asks for help for his student Thorsten, 15 years old, grade 8.

He feels quickly and groundlessly attacked and then fights with his classmates. Since he also aggressively insults teachers with fecal expressions, he has been expelled from the comprehensive school several times and is now in the secondary school as a last chance, although he would certainly meet the requirements of the higher school. The father is very uncooperative, the mother possibly willing to talk. Thorsten himself would like to receive help, as he is unhappy about his uncontrolled aggressions. The school is willing to support Thorsten.

Since Thorsten is a minor, therapy can only take place with the consent of a parent. His mother comes to the conversation only reluctantly—secretly without her husband's knowledge, who would otherwise beat her and Thorsten.

The father is very authoritarian, simply structured, does not tolerate any contradiction. He used to be a boxer and only knows spontaneous harsh punishments and blows as educational methods. The two younger sisters are preferred by him, while Thorsten lives in an unheated shack-like "room", is not allowed to enter the living room, etc. The mother has now resigned and lets her husband have his way. She agrees that her son can come to therapy, but refuses further appointments for fear of her husband. Due to pressure from the school, consultations with a parenting counseling center have already taken place. Because the parents saw Thorsten as the symptom carrier and thus the cause of all problems, they broke off the counseling contacts there.

Since the teachers know the family from other reports, we consider that involving the youth welfare office would with great certainty bring Thorsten blows and could not bring about any changes.

Exploration

Thorsten is very open-minded and wants to stay in school to get a diploma. He often feels attacked very quickly and then thinks that he has to defend himself with aggressive reactions. Only afterwards does he realize how uncontrolled he was and how much he overreacted. He is very unhappy that he rarely succeeds in self-control, which he then experiences not as success, but rather as losing. He cannot give examples of possible or attempted self-control.

Study Questions

- Please consider the genesis of uncontrolled aggressive behavior.
- Consider a therapy plan.
- Which methods of cognitive-behavioral therapy could be combined with hypnosis here?

Diagnosis

It is very clear that Thorsten has not learned to resolve conflicts without violence. In the family, the father's domineering behavior, injustices, etc. always cause an increased level of arousal in Thorsten, which he cannot reduce in the family or through sports. He is therefore always on the defensive and is set on defense (see Sect. 5.2.2). He overvalues small remarks negatively and directed at himself and then reacts uncontrollably and aggressively—as demonstrated at home since kindergarten age.

Clearly, there is model learning here, which also includes low emotional control, frustration tolerance, and self-control.

Prognosis

With the problem that has existed for many years, no changes or improvements are to be seen. The long-standing learning history is based on deficits in self-control, emotional control, etc. The supportive possibilities of the school are limited. Since several school expulsions had to be made due to the aggressions, an intensification of the aggressions must be assumed.

The treatment of aggressions is difficult, as they reduce a pent-up level of arousal, i.e., their negative reinforcement and thus their increase occurs. At the same time, the aggressor is always the center of attention and thereby receives additional operant reinforcement of his behavior, especially when there are large deficits in attention.

In contrast, there is Thorsten's quite large motivation for change, who also cannot expect any help from his family. This led to the decision to give Thorsten a new chance.

Therapy Plan

The widely known relevant training programs for the treatment of aggressions (Petermann 2001) were not yet published at that time and were only for children. The parents' home was not a cooperation partner.

Relatively quick successes had to be achieved, as despite the goodwill of the teachers, further school expulsions could not be avoided in the event of further outbreaks of aggression.

In planning the therapy, it should also be considered that the patient has so far reacted strongly to small triggering stimuli and already lacked regulatory mechanisms. Therefore, a gradual habituation to the previous triggers should take place, combined with concrete instructions for appropriate behavior.

Since the aggressions occurred almost reflexively, counterconditioning could possibly be helpful. At the same time, a new self-regulating behavior had to be built up. With hypnosis, it might be possible to learn new behavior (behavior rehearsal), and in trance then also to effect self-control.

A finger touch on the shoulder as a trigger for the therapy scene should be avoided, as this could easily have been misunderstood by the patient as a physical provocation.

Therapy Implementation

Induction

The induction is done via point fixation, to which he reacts very quickly with relaxation.

Rest Scene

Since he had never traveled before, he finds it difficult to name a beautiful landscape or similar. He spontaneously remembers that he once saw a color postcard of the beach in Ibiza; it was so beautiful that he often raved about it. When he talks about it, it is clearly noticeable how much he mentally and emotionally immerses himself in the scene and will enjoy it in the following hypnosis.

Therapy Scene
He is in hypnosis on the beach of Ibiza, feeling very comfortable and relaxed. Then his teacher appears at some distance and asks him to chatter less (trigger). Now follows the suggestion of the desired alternative behavior: he should smile at her kindly, nod and remain silent (behavior rehearsal, trial action). He succeeds immediately. As a reward, he now receives a large imaginated ice cream with his favorite flavor, which he enjoys (= counterconditioning + positive reinforcement). At the same time, he is praised for his calm behavior, followed by the *posthypnotic suggestion,* to be able to be calm and controlled in similar situations in the future. After the session, he is very surprised about his calm and controlled behavior.

In the next session, he reports that his classmates noticed his calm and appropriate behavior and asked him what was wrong with him. Therefore, he asks not to be quite so calm, as his classmates would otherwise think he was acting. Now the temptation scenes at school become more and more realistic and provocative, as he is in the class, is appropriately criticized and reacts calmly and objectively. Just as I want to switch from external to intrinsic reinforcement, he grins and reports that he has now (in hypnosis) noticed his success, bent down and secretly licked his imagined ice cream under the school desk. It is discussed that he should also reward his successes at school with his imagined ice cream. He also succeeds in this excellently.

After these two to three hypnosis sessions, further support is provided: a conversation is held with the entire class together with the class teacher. For this, I use my TASS method (Training Appropriate School Social Behavior) (Kossak 1978). Since he had so far only received attention for his aggressions in his class, the class is explained to ignore him in case of inappropriate behavior (= withdrawal of reinforcement, extinction, see Sect. 6.1.2, Table 6.1) or to help him become calmer. As soon as he reacts appropriately in critical situations, he receives attention (recognition, pat on the back = reinforcement) from his classmates. They cooperate surprisingly well.

Effects
After a total of ten sessions at increasingly longer intervals, his social behavior, his self-control and his school performance are rated very positively by all teachers. He can stay at this school.

Follow-up
After one year, two and a half and five years, interviews or spontaneous encounters take place. At school, he sometimes only stands out due to slightly disturbed concentration and interjections. When he sees me from his moped, he waves from afar and tells about his development: He completed his school leaving certificate with good grades, is the leader of a scout group at the age of 17, is very socially committed; took up a mechanic's apprenticeship and completed it successfully. He continues to report with joy: When he once kindly asked his father for an increase in pocket money, the father started a physical altercation. Thorsten reacted with

a punch and landed a so-called "lucky punch" that knocked his father out. His mother reacted to this with great amusement. The father recovered, got up and has been cooperative, sociable and kindly pays the increase in pocket money ever since. Thus, the family dynamics spontaneously changed positively. The alpha male stepped back.

Discussion

In the present case, it was not possible to fall back on known or tested therapy measures, especially since the trial period was pressing, during which another school expulsion could occur. A home admission would have become problematic for legal reasons. Since we got along well in the conversations, Thorsten trusted me. Probably this good relationship between us was also a significant therapeutic factor.

The modification of the therapy method makes it clear that beyond the limits of conventional therapy methods, hypnosis can still offer possibilities. His strong calmness and adaptability after the first session is surprising, as this intensity was by no means intended in posthypnotic suggestions. Probably Thorsten experienced the beach scene and the now possible positive reaction possibilities as a relief, which then expressed itself in great calmness.

It is surprising that Thorsten, with this negative educational constellation, did not become antisocial or criminal and was consistently interested in his positive school development, i.e., had performance motivation, possibly resilience. Research on the causes of resilience is still ongoing (Welter-Enderlin 2006).

12.3.15 Case 22—Aggressions After Criminal Influence

Exploration

A young woman, about 22 years old, reacts quickly and uncontrollably with physical aggression for hardly discernible reasons, by aggressively approaching her conversation partners and wanting to hit them. The treating colleague, after several sessions—and knowledge of her life story—agrees with her that she was exposed to an aggressive cult or occult environment for extended periods over the last few years, where strong methods of influence were used on existing or potential members to keep them in the group, so they would adapt to the aggressive rules and vigorously defend themselves against critics and deviants. The patient can hardly defend herself against the sudden fits of aggression, even though she has not been a member of the group for some time. She also does not perceive any triggering causes.

A causal psychiatric background disease for the aggressions could be ruled out.

The colleague now asks for assistance in the case, with the question of whether this behavior could be influenced with hypnosis, as she would like to continue therapy with the patient, but feels potentially physically threatened by her and does not feel up to it. Thus, we conduct the following two sessions together.

Study Questions
- What behavior analysis can you create?
- Please derive a therapy plan from it.

Behavior Analysis
No information is available about the causes of the fits of aggression. Conditioning through post-hypnotic suggestions, using drugs or practices similar to hypnosis, cannot be ruled out.

Prognosis
Given the sometimes very sparse known unfavorable conditions, no particularly favorable prognosis can currently be made, especially since treatment experiences for this problem are not known. This is contrasted by the patient's motivation for therapy, who wants to lead a normal and aggression-free life again. Short-term therapy can only be one module in a long and comprehensive psychotherapy.

Therapy Plan
The attempt should be made to provoke similar aggression-triggering emotions in hypnosis and then interrupt them through suitable interventions and learn self-control. In the case of such strong aggressive actions, in addition to cognitive control, a strong signal for action interruption is also required. This should be done by shouting "Stop". Possibly, the action also needs to be interrupted by the physical intervention of the therapist. If this is successful, the colleague should adopt these methods and include them in her further therapy sessions.

Therapy Implementation

Inductionand Scene of Calm
The patient responds to this relatively quickly and appropriately.

Therapy Scene
A scene is developed in which the patient feels the urge to become tense and aggressive. Unfortunately, we cannot learn anything more about the triggering stimuli or the specifics of the situation. It may be that a general aggression was generated in the "cult scene", which was directed against all persons perceived as "attackers"; a generalization of the aggressions is also to be assumed.

In this scene, she receives—connected with the triggering of the relaxation scene by the wrist touch—the suggestion to hear the word "Stop" and then to become looser and to retreat.

After several repetitions, she can give herself this instruction and we try it in hypnosis. So she gets the instruction to imagine the therapy scene. She then suddenly stands up and then gets the stop instruction. She approaches me quite determinedly. Hears my stop call and only makes physical contact with a bump against the therapist's shoulder.

Effect

Now the *positive suggestions:* "What have you now experienced as positively changed, what is better now!?" are given more often. She cannot verbalize this, but after several of these runs, she reacts more controlled, hesitant, less aggressive. In the next step, the colleague is her practice partner. Initially, the patient is still physically robust, but reacts to the "Stop call", until she can remain looser after several repetitions.

Both the patient and the treating colleague are satisfied with this success, as a more relaxed basis has now been found for further discussions.

Follow-up

The colleague reports weeks after the intervention that the conversations can now proceed more calmly and productively.

In a conversation with the therapist after 19 years, the following can be added. In the further therapy, it was determined that the patient herself was encouraged in the sect to torture and treat people aggressively, which she can hardly or only vaguely remember. In this therapy, the patient's foreign and auto-aggressions became increasingly less. However, she still requires therapeutic support.

Discussion

In this case, we could not identify any triggers of the aggressions, so we could not work causally on it, which was probably also the intention of the perpetrators. Therefore, only direct changes to the symptom were possible in order to reduce conditioned behaviors. As it became clear, this is also possible, but not as quickly and effectively. Here, short-term therapy is only a small, but not insignificant, component in the overall treatment.

12.3.16 Case 23—Self-Efficacy Expectation—Anxiety of the PracticalDriving Test

Exploration

The client (59 years old, divorced) is afraid of her driving test. She passed the theoretical test several months ago, but now, while preparing for the practical test, she is developing increasing fears. After failing the practical test several times, she has become even more uncertain. She has already invested a lot of money in numerous driving lessons and doesn't know what to do.

Upon closer and relaxed exploratory conversation, it becomes clear that she is primarily afraid of the increasing traffic, especially in cities and on the highway. Her aversion to this becomes increasingly evident in her facial expressions and gestures. When suggested to use the traffic practice area with competent accompaniment, she reacts spontaneously with resistance. Finally, she hesitantly admits that she never actually wanted to get a driver's license. But friends and acquaintances pressured her to do so, as it is part of being a modern woman with independence to drive a car.

Study questions

- What do you suggest as the next steps?
- What methodological and content goals should be targeted or achieved?
- What (potential) obstacles can occur?

Diagnosis

This is not a fear in the sense of a phobia, but more about fears of being rejected in her peer group. She experiences a conflict between her own desires "not to drive" and those in her circle of friends "to drive".

Prognosis

Due to the aforementioned conflict, the patient is under high expectation anxiety, which also triggers fears of failure and loss. These can only be successfully reduced by resolving the existing conflict.

Therapy planning, therapy steps

The focus here should be on cognitive restructuring, to appropriately recognize and evaluate the significance of obtaining a driver's license for her personally. The Socratic dialogue is suitable for this (see Sect. 6.1.4), to weigh the pros and cons, fears and emotions, and from this to recognize for herself whether obtaining a driver's license is important to her—or the freedom to experience no pressure and to feel comfortable even without a driver's license.

Therapy implementation

The cautious conversation now aims to learn more about her recognition in these groups, i.e., about her perceived group pressure and her social dependence on the groups. After a short hesitation, she realizes that she has good group contacts and would continue to have her place in the groups even without a car or driver's license.

Thus, the suggestion is made to make a cost-benefit analysis. On the one hand, potential loss of image—on the other hand, costs and effort. So we calculate what further costs she would incur for: driving lessons, examination fees, car purchase, running costs, etc. This is a high sum for her, which makes her thoughtful about wanting to continue to invest so much to be able to drive around at her place of residence and in its relative vicinity. So it is calculated for her that she could spend about 5 € per day on taxi rides in the previously calculated billing period—without fear and excitement. She accepts this argument very relieved, feels visibly relieved, now finally to be able to cope with her own ideas without a car and the associated stress—and to be able to use a taxi with a clear conscience if necessary.

Follow-up
After several months, the client reports in a chance encounter how glad she is to have stopped these tortures of driving lessons and that she can now live as a free person. Certainly, she takes a taxi when needed and enjoys it. She continued to be liked by her friends, etc.

Discussion
The application of short-term therapy for anxiety treatment would not be indicated here. The fear is primarily a cognitive problem, a decision problem. Since she would maintain recognition in her significant reference group even without a driver's license, she is not taking any risk if she does not acquire the driver's license. She realizes that she only wanted to behave according to the anticipated wish of her friends wanted, without checking its reality, which, however, took place in therapy. Since there is still a cognitive dissonance ("I have spent so much money so far—should I continue or stop because of that?"), a very concrete calculation of her future expenses and the resulting gain of being able to afford a taxi more often without losses was made with her. This cost-benefit analysis immediately reduced her cognitive dissonance.

References

Kossak H-C, Zehner G (2011) Hypnose beim Kinderzahnarzt. Verhaltensführung und Kommunikation. Springer, Berlin

Kossak H-C (1978) TASS—Training angemessenen schulischen Sozialverhaltens. Unveröff. Therapiemanual

Kossak H-C (1993) Lehrbuch Hypnose, Kap. 31., 2. überarb u. erw. Aufl., Beltz/PVU, Weinheim

Kossak H-C (2001) Hypnose in der Kinder- und Jugendlichenpsychotherapie. In: Borg-Laufs M (Hrsg.) Lehrbuch der Verhaltenstherapie mit Kindern und Jugendliche. Bd. II: Interventionsmethoden, dgvt-Verlag, Tübingen, S 727–767

Petermann F (1978/2012) Training mit aggressiven Kindern, 13. Aufl., Beltz, Weinheim

Welter-Enderlin R (2006) Resilienz. Gedeihen trotz widriger Umstände. Carl-Auer-Verlag, Heidelberg

Effects, Possibilities of Application, Border Areas

13

Contents

H.-C. Kossak, *Cognitive-behavioral Psychotherapy for Anxiety*,
https://doi.org/10.1007/978-3-662-69099-4_13

13.1 Spontaneous Effects and Side Effects of the Special Short Intervention

13.1.1 Success Stories

Directly after the therapy, that is during the debriefing, patients express their experiences in hypnosis and the entire therapy as follows.

- Immediate, spontaneous, clear positive changes are experienced and reported on all seven levels (of the anxiety components, see Sect. 4.3.2).
- Patients are often amazed and surprised at the rapid and concrete noticeable changes.
- They are particularly surprised and pleased that they have experienced such a change in attitude.
- They are almost always surprised by their newly acquired self-control and self-efficacy.
- At the same time, it is almost self-evident for them to be free from fears from now on and to be able to behave appropriately in the situation as they have always wished.
- After the therapy, patients feel relaxed, relieved, motivated to continue the recommended interventions.

Examples: Statements from Patients

- *"I felt relief, being able to simply look at the object."*
- *"I was suddenly able to act in the situation—just as I always wanted."*
- *"I noticed that I was suddenly able to act again, and the pain then subsided."*
- *"I had to laugh because a simple solution suddenly occurred to me that helped immediately."* ◄

13.1.2 No Side Effects

None of the numerous patients report negative side effects. Even later, after the often experienced euphoria about the positive effects (see above) had subsided and after a greater time distance, no unpleasant side effects of the method were reported.

13.1.3 Impulses from Professional Colleagues

As already mentioned above, I have very often presented this method of short therapy to professional colleagues in seminars at home and abroad and demonstrated it with participants. They presented their relatively multifaceted problems and were very impressed by the short therapy. Also in the subsequent real group exercises with application of the method, they quickly achieved successes. This confirms a quick learnability of the method. At the mentioned congresses, former seminar participants often spontaneously approached me to report their successes with the short therapy method.

Rough Overview of Feedback from Professional Colleagues

- *Age range:* from childhood to old age.
- *Duration:* Is mostly used as short therapy, sometimes also as a module within complex treatments.
- *Indications—Examples:* Fear of cystoscopy, fear of flying, exam anxiety, sleep disorders, professional overload, snake phobia since childhood (afterwards relaxed visit to a market with snakes in Sri Lanka).
- *Evaluation by the patients:* Almost all are very impressed and amazed at the quick effect of the method—and about the impulses in the therapy to be able to evaluate and experience their situation differently (see above).
- *Evaluation by the therapists:* All are amazed and impressed by the mentioned quick and stable effects.
- *Follow-up, relapses:* In the known follow-up periods, the therapy successes remained stable. Neither symptom shifts nor relapses were reported.
- *Effectiveness*: Is rated as high to very high by all therapists and patients.
- *Economy*: Time economy very high, as the method can almost always be successfully completed within one session.

13.2 Modifications of the Method

The approach presented here is almost a standard procedure that was effective in almost all patients in the form presented here. However, depending on the patient and their history or problem situation, modifications of individual therapy parts may be necessary, as also emerged from the case presentations in Chap. 12. Some suggestions for possible modifications of the method follow.

13.2.1 Modifications of Therapy Parts

13.2.1.1 Imagination Problems

If the imagination of scenes is difficult for patients, this can possibly be trained or illustrated with small exercises.

Example: Imagination Exercise

Look at a real apple, then close your eyes and imagine it. Open your eyes and compare the visually perceived real image with the imagination. Then turn the apple in your imagination, feel its weight, smell its typical scent, touch its skin, etc. = VAKOG practice. (For more details see Kossak 2013, p. 347).

Note:

- With such exercises, one usually starts with a simple *image* like an apple. Later, it often develops into a complex *scene*.
- Depending on the imagination "type", sounds, noises are significant for some people, for others colors, movements, etc. Accordingly, the plastic therapist instructions should be aligned. ◄

13.2.1.2 Induction—Difficulties

Some patients require special or individual inductions of hypnosis due to their life history. This will be experienced at the latest when the standard version "point fixation" or "hand levitation" does not work sufficiently or is not accepted. The closer exploration will certainly provide concrete indications of what was perceived as unpleasant. Accordingly, the induction should then be modified.

Sometimes patients want to keep their eyes open for their control. Then the following instruction should be offered at the beginning of the standard instruction (see Sect. 11.1):

"Many patients find closing their eyes pleasant. But if you wish to keep your eyes open, that's also fine. You can decide for yourself whether you want to keep your eyes open or prefer to close them..."

However, the instruction to close the eyes should then be omitted.

13.2.1.3 Rest Scene—Problems, Effectiveness

The rest scene should be carefully explored so that it corresponds to the relaxation wishes of the patient. If, nevertheless, irritations arise during the rest scene, the patient can communicate them so that they can be modified spontaneously.

Example: Rest Scene

- "*I don't want to be near the water ... the calls of the seagulls disturb ...*" accordingly, a change will occur.
- A patient in a group demonstration complained: "*There could be disgusting insects in the meadow.*" He was offered to decide whether he would now prefer to sit in the grass on a blanket. He was able to accept this modification and then enjoy the rest scene.
- A 12-year-old boy gets a severe sneezing fit with a heavily running nose in the deep winter on the "Green Meadow". After immediate termination of the rest scene he reports that he suffers from hay fever. In the previous exploration he had denied the question about hay fever. It had seemed irrelevant to him in winter. Accordingly, the rest scene is changed to an area without potential allergens. This case clearly shows that suggestions trigger imagined scenes that contain classical conditioning reactions. ◄

These examples very vividly show how individual words can trigger complex physiological and immunological reactions.

13.2.1.4 Color Perceptions at the "Negative" and "Positive" Body Site

As illustrated, the patient should touch a body site of well-being according to their therapy phase and alternatively a body site for tension, in order to physically feel the respective associated feeling and thus experience it even more intensely. In some patients, this respective feeling can be intensified if it is associated with another sensory perception. For this purpose, the patient is explored at this point of touch: see the following box.

Example: Modifications—Color Assignment as an Expression of Different Feelings

For the negative feeling of tension or fear, the patient can choose a color that expresses the feeling. This color should then fill the body site and be felt or seen until the switching occurs.

As soon as the relaxation scene is switched to and the patient also places his hand on the responsible site, the patient should imagine the corresponding positive color.

Effects: During the multiple scene changes, the "negative" color is experienced as becoming weaker or it changes towards the "positive" color, until only the positive feeling and the associated color are perceived.

Patients are often very impressed by this clearly "visible" color change, which in turn reinforces the change in behavior. ◀

13.2.1.5 Anxiety Assessment—Scaling

The reactions after therapy are so clearly positive that a strong reduction in anxiety, almost always a complete absence of anxiety, was reported. If you want to be sure as a therapist, you can have the strength of the perceived fear before and after therapy assessed on a so-called SUD scale from 0 (no fear) to 100 (maximum fear) (SUD = Subjective Units of Disturbance).

13.2.2 Modifications of the Therapy Scene

If necessary, the therapy scene can be modified by instructing the patient to experience or carry out changes even more actively *in hypnosis*. Certain methods of VT or hypnosis mentioned below are very helpful in this regard. See also therapy suggestions in Sect. 6.4.2.

Examples: Modifications of Therapy Methods

- *Stimulus Changes:* to experience the previous (acoustic, optical, etc.) triggers for fear as changed or to make the change yourself. Example: Perceiving the fear trigger dog as checkered or with a clown's nose (see case 6) can bring about cognitive restructuring.
- *Observing a Model Person:* The patient observes a person significant to him, who is his role model for fear-free behavior, as she acts in this situation (modelling).
- *Trial Action:* The patient is instructed to try out actions and solutions in hypnosis (behavior rehearsal).
- *Change of Perspective:* To observe oneself from the perspective of another person, acting symptom-related and problem-solving.
- *Age Regression:* In hypnosis age regression, the patient acts as he was able to do successfully in the past (resource activation). ◀

13.3 Considerations on Possible Applications and Boundary Areas

First and foremost, the short form itself should be critically examined.

Preliminary Remark: Limits of the Short Form of Cognitive-Behavioral Hypnotherapy
Especially a short form requires good competencies in order to abstract or compress essential steps from it.

- The short form can tempt to also take a shortened anamnesis and thus only receive superficial, little goal-oriented or even misleading information.
- This can lead to superficial considerations for therapy planning.
- The therapy phase can then be realized too hastily as a quick procedure, incomplete and incomplete.
- "Psychodynamic", hitherto hidden causes, partner problems not mentioned by the patient, childhood trauma, additional burdens (e.g. in smoking cessation, see below) can work in the background and hinder therapy.

13.3.1 Smoking Cessation

The method of short-term therapy was also used by me for smoking cessation.

13.3.1.1 Reaction and Therapy Forms

Broadly classified, two groups can be distinguished in smoking cessation.

13.3.1.1.1 Aversion to Smoking

Depending on the client's wish, the unpleasant smoke and taste of tobacco smoking should be avoided; so he experienced these unpleasant perceptions in hypnosis and could confront them with relaxation, when he self-control with their self-efficacy experienced, thus leaving the unpleasant smoking situation with a good feeling. Accordingly, the posthypnotic tasks are formulated.

13.3.1.1.2 Resisting Temptation Situations

Other clients wanted to be able to resist in the temptation situation, wanting to smoke again. For them, a therapy scene was formulated in which they perceive a certain stimulus, at which they had so far had the desire for a cigarette. This can be the long-conditioned emotional state "stress, cozy, full, anger" or stimulus "seeing a cigarette"—"smelling of tobacco smoke"—"In the pub, at a party" etc.

As soon as the temptation exists to want a cigarette, the client can now interrupt the stimulus effect "desire for a cigarette" by, for example, counteracting with the Everywhere Method, with relaxation counterconditioned and offers alternatives to smoking.

Effects

Many patients already felt relaxed and liberated after this one session, from now on not being situationally dependent on the cigarette. The intervention was able to cause a long to permanent cessation of cigarette smoking in numerous smokers. One client even remained a non-smoker, even though her husband continued to smoke at home.

13.3.1.2 Limits of Smoking Cessation

While the previous success rate of the short-term therapy method for fears was almost 100%, it was about 50% not or only briefly successful for smoking cessation.

The common denominator among clients without treatment success was that all these clients were solely focused on solving their smoking problem and had willfully or unwittingly concealed other problems from me. Once it was the long-standing stress with the girlfriend; in others also partner problems with external relationships and corresponding emotional burdens, up to the impending divorce, the already impending move out of the apartment, etc. In yet another case, the fear of closing doors and the associated fear of flying emerged during the smoker exploration—later, partner problems with the neighbor also emerged here.

My preliminary assumption: Many of these clients wanted to have a justification for now actively working on their problem by registering for smoking cessation—possibly in front of themselves or as an alibi in front of their partner or partner. The improvement of the situation should symbolically take place via the "smoking cessation" and they temporarily had a better conscience.

Self-critical to the method of short-term therapy it is also to be assumed that it is not always specifically aimed at smoking cessation—but why did it then also cause stable and long-lasting successes?

The comprehensive effectiveness of the method for smoking cessation must still be checked.

13.3.2 Impulses for Caution with Very Complex Disorders—Example Test Anxiety

It can certainly happen that one is misled in his causation hypotheses to a disorder; even experienced therapists are not protected from this. The cases cited in the previous chapter with their diagnoses and methodological approaches can therefore only be examples of many possibilities.

As an example of special attention in the anamnesis collection and *possible borderline areas of hypnosis short-term therapy* here—representing many other problem situations—test anxieties are mentioned. Normally, they are very similar and can be successfully treated with relatively simple suggestions in short-term therapy. Some are not clearly delineated; on the other hand, they can manifest themselves in a long chain of causations such as fears, but have profound and long-standing causes in the biography of the person concerned.

13.3.3 Case 24—Exam Anxiety—Lack of Recognition

A professionally active academic has severe learning problems and exam anxieties while studying medicine. He has been struggling with this for many semesters and has only moderate success. Now, close to the final exam, he asks for support. Notable is his extreme avoidance behavior, as he considers every activity more important than studying. It takes weeks of intensive support to properly engage in learning. Eventually, a conversation (despite previous intensive anamnesis) reveals that he never felt accepted by his father, as only the medical exam mattered to him. Therefore, he took up the study of medicine, which he actually did not like and therefore was a torment for him. After his exam, he hopefully will be accepted by his father.

Here, the short therapy method was not applied, but after this realization, an intensive and long therapy was started, which dealt with his relationship with his father. Since the client moved away after passing the medical exam, he committed himself to continue therapy at his new place of residence.

Note

Here it becomes clear that the exam anxiety is real, as the motivation to learn is low. However, the fear of still not being recognized by the father is in the foreground. In this complex case, our short therapy can be little or only punctually helpful as part of a comprehensive therapy.

13.3.4 Case 25—Exam Anxiety—Early Childhood Loss Trauma

The psychology student comes because of exam fears, as she failed in the preliminary diploma examination (today Bachelor) in an oral subject because she hardly spoke anything. The detailed anamnesis reveals: after a social loss trauma in early childhood, the client reacted with mutism: to any demands, especially linguistic ones, she reacted with silence. Therefore, she was almost classified as a dumb special education student.

After an apprenticeship, she passed the high school diploma at night school and studied, always with the self-attribution of actually being a dumb special education student. In the aforementioned exam, she was very hard pressed by the examiner, who was known to be authoritarian, cynical, and misogynistic, with his questions, which she mastered in content. But this situation was a trigger for her childhood mutism.

In numerous therapy sessions, we worked on her childhood trauma, her emotionally cold parental home, etc.—and also with desensitization in hypnosis, to react relaxed to oral demands and to answer accordingly loosely. Her learning for the exam and the various preparations were optimal, so we hardly had to spend time on it. After successfully passing the exam, the entire family problem had to be dealt with, the weight and spread of which only now became apparent, as they were now admitted by the client.

Decades later we met by chance, were happy about the encounter and she introduced herself as a nice and competent colleague.

Note
The exam anxiety here is based on a childhood trauma. It is thus only one aspect of the overall problem of recognition and negative self-evaluation. Accordingly, the fear treatment is also only part of the entire, long and comprehensive therapy.

13.3.5 Case 26—Exam Anxiety—Knowledge Deficits

If a person has large gaps in knowledge, required skills or abilities, then their fear of failing an exam is justified, thus a real fear. It can only be reduced if the gaps are worked through and closed by the targeted acquisition of certain learning and corresponding work techniques etc., including the preparation of written work and preparation of exams (Kossak 2006). If there are still fears, the special method would certainly be helpful.

Note
The therapy here consists, for example, of motivation training, the reduction of external and internal inhibiting factors, and training in relevant learning and work techniques.

13.3.6 Case 27—Exam Anxiety—Fear of Social Negative Evaluation

A student with exam anxiety reports during the anamnesis that he previously underwent group therapy in a therapeutic practice because of his fear. Asked why he now wants individual therapy, he can very hesitantly report that at the end of each group therapy session, everyone was asked in turn what successes or improvements were to report. Since everyone only reported positive things, he was ashamed, simulated improvements, which went unnoticed, and was then discharged as successfully treated. Now in individual therapy, he openly talks about his fears, as he no longer has the fear of negative external attribution. He can be treated with short therapy and passes his exam.

Note
For this student, the fear of negative evaluations and social disregard for deviation due to poor performance is paramount. Accordingly, the fear of negative external attributions was taken into account in the short therapy.

13.3.7 Exam Anxiety—Has Many Subtle and Severe Causes

Diagnosis and Classification of Exam Anxiety are difficult. Synonyms for exam anxiety are: performance anxiety, school anxiety, test anxiety. Its diagnostic classification is also not clear in the DSM-IV diagnostic system and in ICD-10. Accordingly, the clear selection of a therapy is difficult, as is the indication of hypnosis short therapy.

13.3.7.1 Exam Anxiety—At Least Three Symptom Assignments

Exam anxiety can on the one hand be considered a symptom of a *social phobia*, characterized by persistent fear of performance situations or evaluations by other people. However, this only applies to actually socially related areas of fear in exams, such as fear of embarrassing oneself in front of other people.

If an exam (regardless of social evaluations) triggers fear, then it is a "*specific phobia*" of school etc. evaluation situations.

But it can also be a *generalized anxiety disorder* if there is an intense, ongoing worry, associated with fearful expectations, that relates to several events or everyday activities. Since school is of central importance for children, their most common fears relate to homework, classwork, grades, academic success or failure. The same applies to students and learners in general.

Most often a mixed form of all three phobias is found. In younger children, the diagnosis of a specific phobia is very common in the case of exam anxiety.

13.3.7.2 Exam Anxiety as a Borderline Situation

Compared to almost all other aforementioned fears or phobias, real confrontations with the fear situation or the fear trigger can be repeated almost arbitrarily often without affecting further life planning, such as fear of dogs, fear of heights, fear of injections etc.:

- In the case of exams, however, there are clearly defined opportunities for repetition in the event of failure.
- If the exam is not passed after repetitions, the entire previous study is almost meaningless.
- You are then faced with existential questions and fear of the future.
- Therefore, the fear of failing an exam is particularly high.
- Here, the existential fear needs treatment. It must be worked out what alternatives are possible if the last exam opportunity would not be successfully completed.

13.3.7.3 Exam Anxiety as an Expression of, Among Other Things, Fear of the Future

With exam anxiety, it is not necessarily always the fear of failing the exam or of embarrassment that is in the foreground, but the hidden fear of what might come afterwards:

- After several years of enjoying leaving a safe protective framework at the university.
- Transition from freely designed student life to the working world with temporal and content-related demands.
- Leaving a relatively unbound twen and student life—"from free cliffhanger and surfer to tied-up established employee".
- Assumption of far-reaching external responsibility for work, production and personnel.
- Existential fear, no longer being free, having to commit professionally, now being in a phase of life in which one is oriented towards partnership, planning/facing family formation.
- Search for an activity that "is fun", as one is unwilling to endure professional stress and frustration.
- No wonder there is a desire for work-life balance. This is not so unjustified after all …

13.3.7.4 Exam Anxiety—Stage Fright, Performance Anxiety

The fear of public performances as an athlete, musician or actor is associated with special characteristics, as their fear can greatly impair the performance required by the actor.

Examples: Performance Anxiety

The athlete has false starts, the musician stiff fingers or hand tremor, the actor fluffs his lines and his cues. All have in common that they must fulfill a certain timing (at the start, at music cues, role plays) that they cannot influence. With the fear of the performance is usually associated the fear of failure and also the fear of negative criticism, displeasure, career setback etc.

Therefore, with stage fright, the transition to social anxiety, exam anxiety and existential anxiety is fluid. ◄

13.3.7.5 Conclusions on the Indication of the Short Form

These aforementioned profound causes and effects of very different fears can act as causes or contribute to the maintenance of the problem in almost all physical or psychological problems, symptoms, problem situations.

- Therefore, short forms like the one presented here are only designed and successfully applicable for certain areas in diagnostics and therapy.
- They are certainly very helpful as components within a more complex therapy system.

13.4 Impulses from Psychiatry

In the case of *schizophrenia*, a contraindication of hypnosis was often assumed in the past. If the therapist is familiar with this problem and takes into account its own limits and precautions, good results can be achieved with hypnosis, such as for self-control (e.g. Lavoie et al. 1978), even in chronic paranoid schizophrenics (Gafner and Young 1998). Essential are: clarity of images, structuring and emphasis on calm; confusion techniques and indirect techniques are contraindicated (Ebers 1987; Vas 1992).

Maurer (1992) reports on the treatment of fear in a *schizophrenic* who is afraid of hallucinated black holes into which he could fall. Maurer uses behavioral self-control methods.

Heinz (1994) has to admit an *epileptic patient* very often to the hospital because of his seizures, which are often triggered by excitement. In the therapy, posthypnotic tasks are carried out to reduce the excitement through relaxation or to react to the precursors of the seizures with relaxation at the latest, thereby gaining control over the occurrence and frequency of the seizures.

These two *examples for self-control* can serve as an impulse to treat similar psychiatric problem situations also with short-term therapy with hypnosis.

13.5 Extension as a Widely Usable Self-Control Method

All previous clinical examples and areas of application have in common that the presented disorders require a high degree of self-control conviction, self-control, self-regulation and self-efficacy.

Thus, the therapy method required for self-control of anxiety disorders could also be conceivable for the following disorders:

- Improvement of general disease insight and change of lifestyles.
- Adherence to required diet for obesity for weight control and health education (Pittler and Ernst 2005).
- Disorders of impulse control.
- In learning and work disorders cognitive restructuring for setting up and adhering to work plans, work motivation.
- Stress and work management
- Sleep disorders, affective disorders
- Excessive worries and impatience of older people
- Sport: Training support in case of fear of failure, gaining more self-confidence.
- Example diabetes: Weight control and self-control of insulin producing imaginations (Woods and Kulkowsky 1967), as well as changes in attribution for taking self-responsible action (Haisch and Braun 1999) and compliance (Ratner et al. 1990; Blevis et al. 2020; Gonzales et al., 2018; Delamater and Marrero 2020).

The further practical applications will report and decide on this.

References

Blevis L, Gonzales JS, Wagner J (2020) Depression and anxiety in adults with diabetes. In Delamater AM, Marrero AM (Hrsg) Behavioral Diabetes, S 329–352. Springer, New York.

Delamater AM, Marrero AM (2020) Behavioral diabetes. Springer, New York

Ebers W (1987) Überlegungen zum Einsatz von Hypnose bei Patienten mit psychotischer Symptomatik. Experimentelle und Klinische Hypnose 4(2):159–169

Gafner G, Young C (1998) Hypnosis as an adjunct treatment in chronic paranoid schizophrenia. Contemp Hypnosis 15(4):223–226

Gonzales JS, Tannenbaum ML, Commissariat PV (2018) Psychosocial factors in medication adherence and diabetes self-management. Implications für research and practice. Am Psychol 2016 (71):539–551

Haisch J, Braun S (1999) Suggestion von Selbstverantwortung im Rahmen stationärer und ambulanter Diabetikerschulungen. Experimentelle und Klinische Hypnose 15(2):89–104

Heinz A (1994) Hypnose bei einem Patienten mit szenischen Halluzinationen als Aura. Experimentelle und Klinische Hypnose 10(1):3–82

Kossak H-C (2006) Lernen leicht gemacht. Gut vorbereitet und ohne Prüfungsangst zum Erfolg. Carl-Auer, Heidelberg

Kossak H-C (2013) Hypnose. Ein Lehrbuch für Psychotherapeuten und Ärzte, 5. überarb. Aufl., Beltz, Weinheim

Lavoie G, Liberman J, Sabourin M, Brisson A (1978) Individual and group assessment of hypnotic responsity in coerced voluteer chronic schizophrenics. In: Frankel FH, Zamansky SH (Hrsg) Hypnosis at its bicentennial: selected papaers. Plenum Press, New York, S 09–124

Maurer J (1992) Anwendung hypnotherapeutischer Techniken bei schizophrenen Patienten. Experimentelle und Klinische Hypnose 8(1):11–21

Pittler MH, Ernst E (2005) Contemporary therapies for reducing body weight: A systematic review. Int J Obes 25(9):1030–1038

Ratner H, Gross L, Casas J, Castells S (1990) A hypnotherapeutic approach to the improvement of compliance in andolescent diabetes. Am J Clin Hypn 32(3):154–159

Vas J (1992) Hypnotherapie bei Psychosen. Quintessenz, München

Woods SC, Kulkowsky PJ (1967) Classically conditioned changes of blood glucose level. Psychosom Med 38:201–219

14 Cautions, Limits, Contraindications, Effectiveness

Contents

Ultimately, it is important to highlight the application problems of hypnosis and cognitive behavioural therapy (CBT), which may be particularly due to their short form. These include the respective precautions (caveats), limitations, and

H.-C. Kossak, *Cognitive-behavioral Psychotherapy for Anxiety*,
https://doi.org/10.1007/978-3-662-69099-4_14

contraindications. As these are well known from CBT and hypnosis, they are only listed in keyword form below.

Finally, the effectiveness of short-term therapy should be demonstrated, along with an outlook on possible future developments.

14.1 Precautions and Caveats

14.1.1 Consider Possible Basic Problems of the Patient

- Multiple fears can condition each other; they should therefore be addressed individually.
- Pay attention to subjective fear triggers! Only then can successful treatment be possible.
- Make a clear distinction between *problem stimulus* and *relaxation stimulus for relaxation*. Only in this way can the mental and physiological differences be noticed and learned.
- In addition to the emotion "fear", also consider the thoughts, imaginations, evaluations, motivations, and cognitions in their systemic effect and take them into account accordingly (see Chap. 4).
- Depending on the pre-existing problems, close physical proximity of the therapist can be uncomfortable—possibly even contraindicated.
- Choose the most effective relaxation scenes for each individual.

14.1.2 Consider Operant Reinforcements of Fear

- Consider operant learned maintenance of fear through illness gain.
- Include the people in the social system who reinforce the problem in the therapy.
- If there are deficits in attention, the fear symptom as the cause of the attention can be eliminated by the therapy. This results in an additional loss of attention. Accordingly, the patient must receive attention from other sources that reinforce positive problem-solving behaviour. This requires a cost-benefit analysis regarding the attention to be given up and the attention to be gained, etc.
- Operantly maintained fear should only be treated with caution and in relevant sections with the method.
- *In the case of corresponding attention deficits,* the therapist's attention can significantly increase the patient's fear, as he could lose these attentions through healing.

14.1.3 Consider Avoidance Behaviour

- Consider cognitive avoidance behavior such as: distraction, polemicizing. Therefore, for example, do not allow discussions especially in hypnosis.
- Prevent escalations of fear through guidance and possibly through *fractionation,* i.e., interruption of the trance and then continuation with it.
- Always let fear endure before an imagination may be broken off! Otherwise, negative reinforcement occurs, i.e., worsening.
- If the language contact (rapport) is not maintained during hypnosis, the patient can now achieve avoidance with his problem confrontation by deviating into other, harmless imaginations in the best case.

14.1.4 Consider the Reasons Behind the Fear

- To what extent is fear a symptom of avoiding life planning, fear of responsibility, the future with its demands?
- Consider psychodynamic/depth psychologically explainable causes such as early childhood traumas, father issues (see case 24).
- In the case of generalized anxiety disorders and depressions, strong relaxation can lead to brooding and intensive preoccupation with negative thoughts (Kim and Newman 2019).

14.1.5 Can a Later Shoulder Touch Retrigger the Problem Behaviour?

On rare occasions, seminar participants question whether the touch on the shoulder (Phase 6) will continue to be a trigger stimulus for the problem behaviour (fear) after the therapy has concluded. They wonder if an accidental shoulder touch could suddenly retrigger the fear. However, this has never occurred in practice. Through counterconditioning (switching to positive, relaxing imagination, see Sect. 8.3.2), the reduction of avoidance behaviour and the subsequent positive change experiences (Phase 8), the previously triggering effect of the shoulder touch and the subsequent scene (the problem scene) has been completely eliminated. The stimulus has lost its effect and is now perceived neutrally.

14.1.6 Similarity Between Relaxation Scene and Therapy Scene

If the therapy scene and the relaxation scene are too similar, then neither a therapeutic effect nor relaxation can be achieved. Differentiating between a stimulus for relaxation and a stimulus for tension is made difficult by their similarity.

Example: Similar Stimuli Prevent Therapeutic Effect

From a seminar during a partner exercise: The patient is afraid of public speaking; the chosen relaxation scene was the patient giving a humorous speech in a family circle. Here, no emotional differentiation can be made or relaxation achieved, as both scenes contain a speech, i.e., very similar stimuli are present. The relaxation scene "Green Meadow" etc. has a much better relaxation effect for this. ◄

14.2 Limits of the Method

The presented method has all those limits that are generally valid in psychotherapy and hypnotherapy.

- *Unclear genesis of the problem*—requires further exploration.
- *Professional competence* of the therapist.
- *Communication ability* of the patient, e.g., in case of cognitive, social, psychological deficits.
- In case of *fears of losing control* e.g., in psychoses or borderline problems, it should be considered whether individual elements of the therapy can be sensibly used.
- *Excessive self-control*, up to the fear of losing control, loss of reality in hypnosis.
- *Passivity of the patient;* the patient wants solutions without actively working on his problem.
- *Escape from reality* (drugs, addiction, frequent meditation) can possibly be increased by the relaxation in hypnosis.
- *Daydreams* can become compulsive to escape from the outer world of pain or stress or to avoid human interactions (Bigelsen et al. 2016).
- *Fear of hypnosis* in general or specifically, then to blurt out something unwanted etc.—requires intensive clarification and building of trust.
- *Unwillingness of the patient,* to undergo treatment or hypnosis.
- *Low hypnotizability:* then use methods that work solely with imagination. They could be similarly successful.
- *Low imagination ability* can possibly be an obstacle for a hypnosis application. Possibly an imagination training helps here; otherwise, a switch to another therapy method should be made (see Sect. 2.5.2.2.2).

14.3 Contraindications

Here all contraindications apply that are generally valid for the application of hypnosis and CBT. Particularly to be noted are:

- Strong avoidance behaviour
- Rejection of therapy or hypnosis
- Psychodynamic or very complex background of the problem can overwhelm the method. Possibly the overall problem needs to be subdivided for this; possibly the method can be used in partial areas of the problem.

14.4 Effectiveness

14.4.1 Scope and Duration of the Intervention

Previous effectiveness methods, such as stimulus confrontation or desensitization, whether real or in sensu, require substantial preparation and implementation time.

In contrast, short-term therapy sessions typically require only a few scene changes, including those controlled by the patient (phases 2–12). The time required for the entire intervention, excluding exploration, totals between 25 to 40 minutes.

- The method is usually permanently effective after just one session.
- Rarely, and usually only in cases of very severe anxiety problems, are multiple sessions required.

14.4.2 Stability of Behavioural Changes

- Follow-up periods of up to 45 years are available, during which the therapy success remained stable. No known relapses have occurred.
- The behavioural changes are therefore a permanent part of the everyday life of those affected, and are thus resistant to extinction.
- There are no signs of symptom displacement, even though massive cognitive restructurings took place.

14.4.3 Therapeutic Effects

14.4.3.1 Rapid Gain in Autonomy: General and Regarding Profession, Life

Patients are often so impaired by their fears that they may be hindered in their profession or private life, resulting in negative consequences. Through short-term therapy, they can quickly regain their appropriate professional and private life forms without loss.

14.4.3.2 Rapid Change of Reference Systems, Networks etc.

The spontaneous positive experiences of the patient during hypnosis and afterwards clearly indicate that not only a symptom was changed, but a complex reference system of cognitions, attributions etc.

14.4.3.3 Time Economy

The short duration of therapy results in a high degree of time economy. This includes for the patient a treatment as quickly as possible, combined with a rapid gain in autonomy and well-being. Especially with time-bound requirements such as exam fears, interviews or public appearances, a solution can be quickly achieved. Ultimately, this means a reduction in waiting times for therapy practice.

14.4.3.4 Financial Economy

As announced by the Association of Statutory Health Insurance Physicians, short-term therapies are to be remunerated with a bonus (see below).

14.4.3.5 Permanence of Therapy Success—Resistance to Extinction—Follow-ups

The follow-ups clearly show that the therapy resulted in a sustainable and stable change in the reference systems. Its effects are resistant to extinction against previous anxiety-triggering situations or stimuli. The simple experiments from the beginnings of hypnosis and behaviour therapy already proved at that time that the changes in hypnosis remain stable (see Chap. 13, case 25).

14.4.3.6 Generalization

The follow-up questioning of the patients makes it very clear that through short-term therapy not only was fear eliminated and the reference system associated with it changed. Most often, a generalization of self-confident and problem-solving behaviour can be observed, which is also successfully used in other problem situations—including future ones.

14.4.4 Impacts on Psychotherapeutic Practice and Cost Savings

Overall, the extensive and successful case experiences suggest high applicability in psychotherapeutic practice, particularly as in brief therapy. This approach can reduce waiting times, providing quick assistance in cases of significant distress.

The health insurance companies are advocating for cost savings and minimal waiting times.

They particularly favour short-term therapies, offering psychotherapists a 15% surcharge for the first ten sessions with reduced treatment hours (SGB V, 87 paragraph 2c; PTK-Newsletter of the Psychotherapists' Chamber NRW 1/2020).

Furthermore, as of April 1, 2020, the uniform evaluation scale (EBM) of the National Association of Statutory Health Insurance Physicians (KBV) has increased the value of autogenic training, progressive muscle relaxation, and hypnosis by more than 40%.

14.5 Outlook

The effectivity of the method has been successfully determined in over 60 clients. Additionally, a similar number of users, who were seminar participants in Germany and abroad as professional colleagues, have quickly learned and successfully applied this method.

The large and stable success rate should be statistically verified to establish the method as a standard procedure. It is hypothesized that the method is effective not only in cases of anxiety disorders, such as in situations of temptation (eating disorders, diet for diabetics, smoking), but also for the intervention in and self-control of pain attacks, aggressions, and epileptic seizures. It is likely that appropriate modifications of this short form are also effective in learning and work disorders and "simple" exam anxieties.

References

Bigelsen J, Lehrfeld JM, Jopp DS, Somer E (2016) Maladaptive daydreaming: Evidence for an under-researched mental health disorder. Conscious Cogn 42:254–266

Kim H, Newman MG (2019) The paradox of relaxation training: Relaxation induced anxiety and mediation effects of contrast avoidance in generalized anxiety disorder and major depressive disorder. J Affect Disord 259:271–278

Newsletter der Psychotherapeutenkammer NRW, 1/2020

Further or Supplementary Literature by the Author on the Subject of Hypnosis in Combination with Cognitive-Behavioural Therapy

The literature may possibly suggest delving more into hypnosis, possibly even with the combination of cognitive-behavioral therapy and hypnosis.

Kossak H-C (1985) VT – Verhaltenstherapie unter Hypnose. Selbstkontrolltraining mit dem „hypnotischen Begleiter". Experimentelle und klinische Hypnose 1(2):113–142

Kossak H-C (1987) Verhaltenstherapie nächtlicher Asthmaanfälle. Kognitive Umstrukturierung unter Hypnose. Hyp Kognit 4:41–57

Kossak H-C (1990a) VT – Behavior therapy and hypnosis: Methods of self-management. Kongressvortrag und Seminar. 5th European Congress of Hypnosis in Psychotherapy and Psychosomatic Medicine. Konstanz

Kossak H-C (1990b) Verhaltenstherapeutische Selbstkontrolle unter Hypnose. Verhaltensther & Psychosoziale Praxis 2(90):199–224

Kossak H-C (1991a) Hypnose. Modetrend oder berechtigte Renaissance. Psychomed 3(3):150–155

Kossak H-C (1991b) Fallbeschreibung: Brechdurchfälle, Depressionen und Examensprobleme. In: Peter P, Kraiker C, Revenstorf D (Hrsg) Hypnose und Verhaltenstherapie. Hans, Bern, S 81–92

Kossak H-C (1991c) Hypnose-Behandlung bei Colitis ulcerosa – Ein Fallbericht. Psychomed 3(3):170–171

Kossak H-C (1992a) Verhaltenstherapeutische Selbstkontrolle durch Hypnose bei schulischen Lern- und Leistungsstörungen – Fallbericht. Experimentelle und Klinische Hypnose 8(1):23–42

Kossak H-C (1992b) Behavior therapy and hypnosis: methods of selfmanagement. In: Bongarzt W, Bongartz B, Gheorghiu V (Hrsg) Hypnosis: 175 years after Mesmer. Recent developments in theory and application. Proceedings of the 5th European Congress of Hypnosis, S 189–199

Kossak, H-C (1994) Selbstmanagement-Therapie unter Hypnose. Sexueller Missbrauch oder stellvertretende Ängste. Fallbericht. Experimentelle und klinische Hypnose 10(1):1–22

Kossak H-C (2001) Hypnose in der Kinder- und Jugendlichenverhaltenstherapie. In: Borg-Laufs M (Hrsg), Lehrbuch der Verhaltenstherapie mit Kindern und Jugendlichen. Dgvt, Tübingen, S 727–767

Kossak H-C (2008) Ängste im schulischen Lern- und Leistungsprozess und bei Prüfungen. Ganzheitliche Diagnostik und Therapie – Impulse aus der Praxis für die Praxis. Zeit-schrift für integrative Lerntherapie, 8(2), Beitrag auf CD. Zeitschrift für Integrative Lerntherapie, Heft 2. auf CD.

Kossak H-C (2009a) Aversive Handlung endlich beginnen. In: Fliegel S, Kämmerer A (Hrsg) Psychotherapeutische Schätze II. dgvt, Tübingen, S 27

H.-C. Kossak, *Cognitive-behavioral Psychotherapy for Anxiety*,
https://doi.org/10.1007/978-3-662-69099-4

Kossak H-C (2009b) Erfolg vorwegnehmen und dann endlich handeln. In: Fliegel S, Kämmerer A (Hrsg) Psychotherapeutische Schätze II. dgvt, Tübingen, S 63

Kossak H-C (2009c) Roter Ballon. In: Fliegel S, Kämmerer A (Hrsg) Psychotherapeutische Schätze II. dgvt, Tübingen, S 157

Kossak H-C (2009d) Weggabelung zur Entscheidung. In: Fliegel S, Kämmerer A (Hrsg) Psychotherapeutische Schätze II. dgvt, Tübingen, S 200–202

Kossak H-C (2011) Hypnose. In: Linden M, Hautzinger M (Hrsg) Verhaltenstherapiemanual, 7. Aufl. Springer, Berlin, S 175–181

Kossak H-C (2014) KVT und Hypnose: Die Rekonstruktion, Konstruktion und Bearbeitung problemrelevanter Kognitionen in Hypnose. In: Stavemann HH (Hrsg) KVT-Praxis. Strategien und Leitfäden für die Integrative KVT, 3. Aufl. Beltz, Weinheim, S 648–673

Kossak H-C (2015) Patienteninformationen zur Hypnose. In: Stavemann HH (Hrsg) Therapie-Tools. Integrative KBT. Beltz, Weinheim, S 548

Kossak H-C (2020) Hypnose. In: Petermann F, Vaitl D (Hrsg) Entspannungsverfahren, 5. Aufl. BeltzPVU, S 99–115

Made in the USA
Monee, IL
13 September 2026

62973765R00155